Care and Respect in Bioethics

Care and Respect in Bioethics

By

Darlei Dall'Agnol

Cambridge
Scholars
Publishing

Care and Respect in Bioethics

By Darlei Dall'Agnol

This book first published 2016

Cambridge Scholars Publishing

Lady Stephenson Library, Newcastle upon Tyne, NE6 2PA, UK

British Library Cataloguing in Publication Data
A catalogue record for this book is available from the British Library

ISBN (10): 1-4438-9783-3
ISBN (13): 978-1-4438-9783-9

To Juliana:
with care + respect = love.

While the ethics of rights is a manifestation of equal respect, balancing the claims of other and self, the ethics of responsibility rests on an understanding that gives rise to compassion and care. Thus, the counterpoint of identity and intimacy that marks the time between childhood and adulthood is articulated through two moralities whose complementarity is the discovery of maturity.
—Gilligan

TABLE OF CONTENTS

ACKNOWLEDGMENTS

This book presents the results of my work in bioethics over the past eight years. The idea was born in May 2007 when I read the paper "Care & Respect in Medicine" at the faculty seminar "Bioethics, Values & Society" in the Medical School of the Health System at the University of Michigan, US. I was in Ann Arbor doing post doctorate research under Professor Stephen Darwall's supervision, and I wanted to develop the project of a new moral epistemology, namely practical cognitivism, which will become apparent here. The suggestions and criticism of Susan Goold, Mike Fellters, Maria Silveira and David Shalowitz led me to plan an extended work. This is it.

At that time, I was focusing mainly on meta-ethical issues, but I then came across Darwall's theory of rational care, which I will reconstruct later, and started to ponder its implications for bioethics, especially whether it was able to avoid some forms of paternalism, a topic I discussed with Darwall several times. Thus, I got the idea of 'respectful care' through conversations with Darwall, and I am in debt to him for much of the inspiration for this work. I would also like to thank Peter Railton for our discussions in Ann Arbor and in Florianópolis, especially for his encouragement to develop a new moral epistemology based on the idea of *knowing-how* to ground respectful care.

In 2009, I spent four months at Michigan State University, in East Lansing, a well-known place for bioethical studies mainly from a feminist point of view. There I read the paper "Care & Respect" (now published in *Bioethikos*) in a joined section of the Center for Ethics and Humanities in the Life Sciences and the Department of Philosophy, and the contributions of the audience, especially those of Hilde Lindemann and Jamie Nelson, were important in expanding the work to include care ethics. I will discuss some of their ideas throughout this book. In East Lansing, I completed a first draft of this book, and I am grateful to Professor Frederick Rauscher for our philosophical conversations during this time and afterwards, especially on the extent and limits of the Kantian principle of respect for persons.

Back in Brazil, I continued thinking about the meta-ethical and normative bases of bioethics, but my teaching duties and my role as the

Director of the Graduate Programme in Philosophy at the Federal University of Santa Catarina forced me to put the book to one side for a while. Despite this administrative function, I had the opportunity to discuss some parts of this work with Brazilian colleagues at many conferences. Thus, I would especially like to thank Dr. Marco Azevedo for his critical comments on the first draft. Thanks also to the graduate students who contributed to my work; I will not mention names here since I fear leaving many out. I would also like to thank the editors of *Bioethikos* for authorizing the publication of parts of my paper "Cuidar & Respeitar: atitudes fundamentais na bioética," in which I first presented the idea of respectful care in print.

In 2012, I went to Georgetown University for the 38th IBC – Intensive Bioethics Course. I felt that I had to learn the basics of the predominant bioethical theory in Washington. Thus, I would like to thank Carol Taylor and Maggie Little for our discussions on the normative foundations of bioethics. I owe to Carol an interesting and updated reading of the so-called "principlism" or "the four principles approach" (*respect for autonomy*, *non-maleficence*, *beneficence* and *justice*), the Georgetown Mantra. I would also like to thank Maggie Little for her important input on the epistemology to ground respectful care. I will discuss Little's particularist interpretation of Wittgenstein's ethics as well as casuistry and other relativistic views throughout this work. The discussion of the meta-ethical and normative bases of bioethics is here centred around principlism. Basically, I criticise the intuitionist meta-ethics of principlism substituting it for practical cognitivism in proposing a new bioethical concept, namely respectful care. I got this idea during the 38th IBC.

In its final form, this book is the result of a sabbatical year and my research carried out as a Visiting Scholar at the Uehiro Centre for Practical Ethics, at the University of Oxford, UK, in 2015. Thus, I would like to thank especially Professor Roger Crisp for supervising my work, Dominic Wilkinson for our conversations on the normative foundations of neonatal bioethics and Julian Savulescu for his constant support. The idea of respectful care was published in English on Uehiro's blog *Practical Ethics in the News* together with associated posts such as "caring robots", "caring for our home" and "enhancing wisdom" (see: http://blog.practicalethics.ox.ac.uk/darlei-dallagnolls-posts/), which are parts of chapters of this book. I would like to thank the Uehiro Centre for authorizing the use of this material. I would also like to thank the *Journal of Medical Ethics* (v.42) for authorizing the publication of an extended version of my essay "Knowing-how to care," which is now part of this work (chapter 5), that is, the bulk of this book.

I benefitted also in writing the final version from some suggestions made by Frederick Rauscher and Roger Crisp. I could not, however, respond to all their comments and I apologise in advance for the remaining mistakes. I would finally like to thank Kim Butson for helping revise the grammar. Last, but not least, thanks to CAPES and CNPq, two Brazilian federal agencies, for providing financial support for my research over the years.

INTRODUCTION

This is a work on the *philosophical* foundations of bioethics. The main problem it deals with is related to the tensions and potential dilemmas generated by the intuitionist meta-ethical commitments of the predominant normative theory, namely "the four principles approach" (also known as "principlism"). This view is based on the *prima facie* norms of respect for autonomy (*one ought to respect the autonomous choices of subjects of scientific research/patients*), non-maleficence (*one ought to refrain from inflicting harm*), beneficence (*one ought to do good and prevent or remove harm*) and justice (*one ought to treat people fairly*). I will examine this approach in greater detail in chapter 3. The tensions in applying these basic principles may lead to inaction in scientific experiments involving human subjects or to arbitrary applications of the norms in the art of caring. My main goal is then to find a proper balance between caring & respecting at the normative foundations of bioethics. The problem can be made explicit in these terms: on the one hand, caring without respecting seems blind, degenerating into forms of paternalism when, for instance, the one-caring imposes her conception of the good life or a particular procedure on the cared-for; on the other hand, respecting without caring amounts to indifference or individualism when, for example, a person does not look after a vulnerable being properly. The question then is: how can we avoid both paternalism and indifference in caring & respecting?

My initial hypothesis is that the concept of *respectful care* can be built up, working from an ethico-philosophical perspective, to be a leading notion capable of guiding our daily actions and bioethical practices. This concept has the potential to overcome the problematic intuitionist meta-ethics of the predominant normative theory in bioethics. In order to show this, I will formulate a new moral epistemology, practical cognitivism, to give support to the concept of respectful care and, consequently, to provide better bases for bioethics. To recognize its plausibility, I will illustrate how it might work in *a* common, sharable morality, paying particular attention to bioethical cases in the neonatal context. I will then argue that a respectful caring manner may be considered one of the most fundamental *attitudes* we must cultivate in all domains of our moral lives. I will exemplify its implications particularly in the field of bioethics because this moral domain raises issues that concern us all, such as whether we should edit the human genome to avoid disabilities using CRISP-Cas9, whether abortion is morally permissible, whether we should be assisted in dying etc. Respectful care is not only undoubtedly important in scientific research involving human subjects, especially in the health care system, but also in all domains of our daily lives.

I will, methodologically speaking, use conceptual analysis as an important philosophical tool. That is to say, I will *search* for the conditions (I hope the necessary and sufficient ones) under which we apply correctly a word, an expression etc. as it was put forward, for instance, by Nel Noddings in her book *Caring* (p.69): "logically, we have the following situation (W, X) is a caring relation if and only if:

i) W cares for X (as described in the one-caring) and
ii) X recognizes that W cares for X."

Noddings' analysis does not seem right to me as some conditions are not necessary at all (e.g., the cared for does not need to recognize that the one caring is looking after her), and even if they were, they would conjointly not be sufficient. Moreover, her analysis seems circular: she cannot use the *analysans* "cares for" to clarify the *analysandum* "caring relation". Thus, I will look for a better one, without pretending to offer a final analysis, especially in terms of a *respectful* caring attitude and apply it using concrete, practical bioethical cases. My analysis of knowing-how to care respectfully will try to overcome the difficulties generated by the intuitionist meta-ethics of principlism. In this sense, the general aim of this book is to rethink the meta-ethical and normative bases of bioethics in order to offer a better alternative to the predominant approach.

In order to achieve this general goal, I will, in the first chapter, reconstruct the main tensions and apparent dilemmas between caring & respecting (section 1.1) in the domain of what can be called "special bioethics", that is, the ethical problems involved in doing research using human subjects in, especially but not restricted to, the biomedical sciences. To illustrate such problems, I will tell the story of Baby 1 showing why the predominant bioethical approach apparently fails to give a proper solution to the ethical problems of the case. I will then, in section 1.2, discuss the need for both a new concept in special bioethics to avoid the problems and an innovative moral epistemology to ground it, two tasks a solid *philosophical bioethics* must be capable of accomplishing.

In the second chapter, I will start to scrutinize some of the meta-ethical commitments of the predominant approach beginning with the supposed consensus reached around the Belmont Report (US, 1978), when bioethicists of different ethical traditions, namely casuists, utilitarians, deontologists, etc. reached a "compromise" on basic principles for research involving human beings. This report gave rise to principlism. Thus, in section 2.1, I will discuss methodological questions such as whether we should work with cases only, as the commissioner and philosopher Albert Jonsen argued in cooperation with Stephen Toulmin; or with universal principles too, as the principlists Tom Beauchamp and James Childress held later. I will, in section 2.2, make a detailed reconstruction of the three basic principles of the Belmont document, namely *respect for persons*, *beneficence* and *justice*.

In the last forty years of bioethical discussions, there have been two main departures from the Belmont framework, which I will examine in the third chapter. First, in their now classic book *Principles of Biomedical Ethics*, Beauchamp and Childress argued that we should work with *four* principles instead, dismembering non-maleficence from beneficence, and that a basic norm is respect for *autonomy* and not respect for *persons*. They kept, however, the intuitionist meta-ethics of the document. I will discuss their principlist views, which became predominant, in section 3.1. Second, both Tristam Engelhardt and Edmund Pellegrino have tried to overcome the problems generated by the four principles approach by ranking *one* basic norm over the others and, in this way, abandoning the intuitionist meta-ethics. Thus, I will, in section 3.2, discuss these solutions, which lead to *autonomism* and *the beneficence-in-trust model*. To point out the problems of these approaches, I will introduce the case of Baby 2 arguing that we should look for a better way of integrating care & respect into a coherent whole leading to the idea of respectful care as the core concept for *a* common, sharable morality.

In the fourth chapter, I will scrutinize the idea of *the* common morality used by the principlists to ground bioethical decisions. I will, in section 4.1, make a reduction of the principles of respect for autonomy and justice re-analysing the idea of *respect* for a person's rights. Moreover, I will reduce the principles of non-maleficence and beneficence to *care* also re-analysing this concept in order to point out a way of integrating care & respect into the concept of respectful care. As we will see, these are the main cornerstones of *a* common, sharable morality. To illustrate how this might work, I will, in section 4.2, discuss end-of-life care, especially whether we should kill or let die premature babies with no prospect of cure. As we will see, taking a life can paradoxically be seen as an expression of compassionate care. That is to say, we must *know-how* to care in a proper way.

In the fifth chapter, I will then present the main tenets of a new moral epistemology, namely practical cognitivism, to give support to the idea of respectful care. I will do this mainly in section 5.1. In order to achieve this goal, I will introduce the case of Baby 3 showing what care without respect amounts to. In the second part (5.2), I will finally propose a conceptual analysis of knowing-how to care respectfully sorting out the necessary and, I hope, sufficient conditions to apply this fundamental bioethical notion. This will, I believe, be the main contribution of this book.

In the next chapter, I will go back to the cases of Baby 1, Baby 2 and Baby 3 considering what would have been the right course of action had the concept of respectful care been taken seriously. These bioethical cases are just illustrations of how respectful care might work. They will be discussed in section 6.1. Moreover, I will, in section 6.2, argue that one of the central roles of bioethics committees is to guarantee that respectful care is always in place in our daily acts and bioethical practices.

Finally, I will consider how respectful care may be extended to other bioethical domains, especially to what can be called "global bioethics" (the discussion of bioethical issues in the international arena) and "holistic bioethics", that is, caring for life as a whole including the environment and non-human animals. As an illustration, and to keep an eye on the future, I will speculate what a respectful caring robot may look like in section 7.1. Some bioethical issues related to the original idea of bioethics as a concern for life as a whole will be discussed in section 7.2. The integration of "special bioethics" with "global bioethics" and "holistic bioethics" is realised by the idea of a *philosophical* bioethics.

The justification for this work can be put in very simple terms: bioethics deals with questions of life and death that concern us all, so it is crucial to get its meta-ethical and normative foundations right. To know-how we must live (and die) is no trivial issue. In fact, I know of no more important matter.

CHAPTER ONE

CARE *VERSUS* RESPECT

To start with, I would like to sort out in greater detail the background *problem* I am trying to present a solution to here. Caring for and respecting someone are, according to some current (bio)ethicists, two ways of intrinsically valuing an individual and/or a person. For this reason, they are frequently considered fundamental moral and bioethical notions, and it seems natural to assume that they would form a harmonic whole guiding our moral lives, our everyday actions such as looking after our children or caring for non-human animals and also most of our complex practices, for instance, doing biomedical research and scientific experimentation on vulnerable patients. In other words, they appear to complement each other. Common sense or sound judgment seems to tell us that this is really the case. However, these moral notions may also clash with each other and even stand in opposition generating tensions, conflicts and dilemmas, which may ultimately lead to inaction. Most forms of paternalism, that is, the intentional overriding of a person's preferences and values with the goal of supposedly benefiting her, are disrespectful.

These tensions are sometimes cast in the following languages:

i) attempts to foster collective wellbeing or the welfare of a given community *versus* accepting individual preferences;
ii) the long Hippocratic tradition in medicine requiring us first *to care for* the patient *versus* a modern morality that demands first *respect for* the patient's lifestyle, values and choices;
iii) the responsibilities of doctors and/or researchers in their dual roles as scientists and as physicians in biomedicine *versus* the rights of the subjects of scientific experimentation;
iv) a female moral voice supposedly based on personal commitments and sentiments *versus* a male morality allegedly based on impartial rights and principles of justice;
v) the particular requirements of contextualized caring *versus* universal values based on respect.

I will argue in this work that these tensions do not lead to *real* moral dilemmas or even to opposite moralities and that most conflicts can be resolved.

These tensions are not bad in themselves (as they are not in music, in love or in many other domains of human life) and may even perform a creative role, but they certainly call for a resolution. The dialectical contrast between opposites may generate harmony, but the tensions between caring & respecting can also lead to inaction if they are not solved or dissolved. It might be the case that care & respect stand for two opposite poles in our moral lives and that they limit each other creating a harmonic whole. That is to say, it seems to be the case that respect *limits* care, avoiding it turning into paternalism; and that a caring attitude complements respect, escaping indifference or individualism. Consequently, finding the right equilibrium between caring & respecting is nowadays one of the main challenges in philosophical ethics, and it constitutes the main ambition of the present work.

Some important bioethical questions then are these: is it really possible to reach a right balance between caring & respecting? How can we regard them as interconnected, as mutually supporting attitudes capable of overcoming the above mentioned dichotomies? Are they in fact incompatible and, for instance, respect for a patient's autonomy must always *trump* welfare concerns when they conflict? To give an illustration: what about a patient's request (or from her proxy/surrogate) for an *experimental* drug or some medical procedure that offers no clear benefit and may even cause potential harm, is a health professional under the obligation to provide it? If not, does that not constitute negligence or malpractice?

In this chapter, I will reconstruct in a more detailed way how caring & respecting may conflict and start to look for a resolution of these tensions. In the first section, I will present a particular case to illustrate how care may not always be accompanied by respect. In the second section, I will propose the idea of bioethics guided by philosophical *wisdom*, which can be defined in terms of knowing-how to live well, as a discipline capable of integrating caring & respecting into a coherent whole in our moral lives.

1.1 Caring and disrespecting

In order to illustrate at once the complex imbrications between caring & respecting, let me introduce a particular bioethical case involving, on the one hand, health professionals, researchers (some in fact with dual roles), students etc. and, on the other hand, a very special patient, an extremely-premature baby, who happened to be in a circumstance where she could also be the subject of experimental scientific research in a teaching hospital. Consider then the following real life case, reconstructed here in the Hastings Center Report's style, which does not imply that I am assuming a casuistic-based approach to bioethical problems:

> Baby 1 was born prematurely (23 weeks), on 07/15/2006, Michigan, US. She weighed 1 pound and 5 ounces and was 11 3/4 inches long. Baby 1 belonged to the Extremely Low Birth Weight (ELBW) group of babies. She had small haemorrhages in her brain and respiratory failure. On 08/04/2006, she was transferred to another NICU (Neonatal Intensive Care Unit) because she required surgical placement of a ventricular reservoir to relieve pressure on the brain caused by bleeding. Because of her immature lungs, she breathed with the aid of a ventilator and was receiving morphine to relieve pain. She had infections and was on antibiotics. On 09/01/2006, she was diagnosed with a potentially fatal intestinal disease, namely NEC (*Necrotizing Enterocolitis*) which causes bowel tissue to die. She could not survive and was expected to live 2 days more. The parents agreed that *palliative care* only was appropriate and prepared themselves for the worst. After 2 weeks, however, the baby was still alive and being kept comfortable with sugar water and potassium, but with no nutrition at this time (and surprisingly) *against* the wishes of the parents. A suit was filed on 09/15/2006 against the U. of A. (the hospital's fictional name here) naming the Regents, 4 physicians and other staff as defendants. The parents went to court arguing that only they had the right to decide whether life sustaining treatment should be given or withheld. Meanwhile, a second opinion was sought. Some hospitals were apparently willing to accept a transfer (e.g., Toledo Children's Hospital), but they made clear that they probably couldn't do better than the U. of A. Besides, the parents' health insurance would not cover the transfer. The Ethics Committee of the U. of A. decided, in any case, that Baby 1 should not be transferred. An intestine transplant was also considered (at Children's Hospital of Pittsburgh), but the responsible paediatric surgeon decided that no further treatment was appropriate since the arteries that normally supply blood to the intestines were clotted and useless. Just one night before the court hearings, which could have ordered the hospital to increase care, Baby 1 passed-away (09/19/2006).

These are some of the basic *facts* of the case; other facts and some ethical reflections will become apparent throughout this book. Note, however, that I am distinguishing scientific *facts* from *values*, which will be discussed below. We need to do that not only to provide a proper solution to the case, but also in order to avoid conflating scientific issues with ethical ones.

Take another look at the picture on the cover of this book. Preterm babies in these conditions are in a very fragile, extremely vulnerable state. This is perhaps the plainest example of the *vulnerability* of the human condition and of the unquestionable fact of *our mutual interdependence*. No doubt, Baby 1 needs attention, but *how* best to care for her? The blue plastic tube is the ventilator, attached to a computer that regulates the speed at which she breathes and the percentage of pure oxygen in each of those breaths. The round patch stuck to her chest is to measure her heartbeat. The needles in her arms provide medication and nutrition. The thin wires are threaded into an umbilical artery and vein to give intravenous fluids. The patches over her eyes protect from blindness etc. We are no doubt care-dependent creatures. A crucial ethical question is this: are we not *disrespecting* Baby 1?

There are other questions: should we use technology just because it is available even if it produces more harm than good, that is, should we follow the technological imperative ("what *can* be done, *must* be!")? Perhaps the central question is whether technicized medicine is not doing too much and thus causing more harm than good. So, when is enough really enough? Why should we not allow a baby in this condition to die in peace before starting any lifesaving support? Is euthanasia morally permissible? Why not euthanize Baby 1 instead of withdrawing food, just because the parents have strong religious values? But should doctors' decisions be bound by religious beliefs? Is there a background conflict between a scientific and a religious worldview in this case, if so, which should prevail?

The predominant normative theory in bioethics, namely the four principles approach, based on the *prima facie* norms of respect for autonomy, non-maleficence, beneficence and justice, which will be examined soon in greater detail (section 3.1), apparently fails to give a proper solution in this case. That is to say, it in no way tells us whether we should *respect* the parents' request to increase care or accept the doctors' prognosis that palliative *care* is the only course of action morally and technically recommended. It has no clear criterion to apply either the principle of respect for autonomy *or* the principle of beneficence. This is even recognized by the main proponents of principlism: "These conflicts sometimes produce irresolvable moral dilemmas."[1] Now, a moral dilemma is a situation where an agent is under two obligations, but it is impossible

---

[1] Tom L. Beauchamp and James F. Childress, *Principles of Biomedical Ethics*, (New York/Oxford: Oxford University Press, 2013), 12.

to perform both duties. Moral dilemmas, however, may not be real.[2] Most likely, they are only *apparent* given the epistemic limitations of the agent. They cannot anyway be generated by the bioethical theory itself. This is unacceptable and shows that the predominant bioethical theory seems flawed. How did we come to such a state of affairs in bioethics, including in the neonatal context?

In order to answer this question, we need perhaps to understand better the development of this particular science, namely neonatology, and its *moral* challenges. It can generally be defined as the science of the diagnosis and treatment of disorders that affect newborns. Neonatology, which provides high-intensive care to premature infants, is one of the most technically sophisticated areas of medicine. It is fascinating, but it also deals with hard moral cases. It can be an aggressive, intrusive branch of medicine. Paediatricians may do everything within their power to keep, so to speak, this "patch of flesh alive." As the present story of Baby 1 shows, moral dilemmas concerning the choice between saving the patient or letting her die may be routine. New technologies have made it possible to save the lives of infants who only a few years ago would certainly have died. We can, for instance, recall here that the surfactant (for example, poractant alpha), which coats the tiny air sacs of the lungs, is a recent scientific discovery. This is a fine example of how science can work for our benefit, to increase our wellbeing. Without it, Baby 1 would not have survived the day she was born. There is little doubt then that the sciences and technology can be used for our own good. We need to ask, however, ethical questions as well: what about the consequences of the treatment, for instance, will the baby suffer from a severe intellectual disability or any other impairment later in life? Should we save her or let her die? There is no easy answer to this latter question. As can be seen, moral dilemmas are still very common in this medical area as the Baby 1 case clearly shows.

To find out what went wrong in Baby 1's case, we also need to present some developments in neonatal bioethics. That is to say, her story needs to be seen in the context of developing new treatments in neonatology and the *moral* challenges this brings. Now, according to Lantos and Meadow,

[2] As Tristram Engeldhart wrote (*The Foundations of Bioethics,* New York/Oxford: Oxford University Press, 1996, 103): "This tension can be appreciated as the conflict between two ethical principles: that of permission and that of beneficence." Now, if one gives always absolute priority to permission, then the tensions disappear and there is no *real* dilemma. I will discuss Engelhardt's solution later.

the development of neonatology in the past decades has gone through three different eras:

i) *the era of innovation and individualism* (1965-1982). This era began with the introduction of mechanical ventilation for premature babies and was driven by the technological imperative, which meant that whatever could be done to save the babies' lives ought to be done;
ii) *the era of exposed ignorance* (1982-1992). This era began with a controversy over a case, namely Baby Doe, who was allowed to die rather than undergo lifesaving surgery. During this era the paediatricians and neonatologists began to face criticism for inappropriately withholding treatments that parents might have wanted. There was no consensus about what ought to be done in most cases, that is, doctors did not know how to apply the Baby Doe guidelines;
iii) *the end of medical progress* (1992 to the present). The end of medical and technical progress in neonatology had important moral implications. Researchers asked parents what they really wanted.[3]

These eras reveal the tensions between the technological imperative and moral ignorance or, at least, moral uncertainty. There is no easy answer, but we certainly need to do better.

I would now like to call attention to two points. First, note that, in the second era reconstructed above, doctors did not *know how* to apply specific guidelines. That is why we certainly need a new moral epistemology, as I will argue soon. Second, in the third era, autonomy apparently became the first principle of bioethics overriding all others. Now, giving "parents what they really want" seems no solution at all. Is it right to say that the principle of autonomy, which will be analysed later in detail when discussing autonomism (section 3.2), is the supreme norm of neonatal bioethics? Is it morally right to give the parents of Baby 1 what they actually want even if this disrespects her as a person or is against the Hippocratic moral tradition based on the principle of non-maleficence? Again, it seems that principlism cannot help us out of these tensions; we need to do better. For this reason, I believe we must develop a new moral epistemology grounding morality on *knowing-how* (e.g., to care respectfully) to overcome this state of "exposed ignorance". I hope to

[3] John D. Lantos and William L. Meadow, *Neonatal Bioethics*, (Baltimore: The John Hopkins University Press, 2006), 18f.

make a contribution to leaving behind this state of affairs with the concept of respectful care based on a new moral epistemology, namely practical cognitivism.

Let me now make another methodological point concerning bioethical investigations right at the beginning of this work. Starting with a case as I did (and I will present others soon) does not imply that I am subscribing to a particularist ethical approach, which denies that there are universal principles. As Hilde Lindemann correctly puts it: "It is often assumed that, when an ethicist works with cases, they are taking a narrative approach to clinical ethics. In this essay, I argue that this is typically not true …".[4] Thus, I do not intend to do *narrative* ethics or assume any other "bottom-up" particularistic approach to ethics at this point, that is, work from particular cases to general norms. I will follow, however, *some* casuist methodological advice, for instance, discussing real-life cases instead of fictional ones. I will not defend casuistry, which is only committed to *general* norms in analysing paradigmatic cases. On the contrary, I will try to show throughout this work that any bioethical case must be approached with clear moral *universal* principles at hand. I will return to this point later. Consequently, I take particular bioethical cases only as illustrations of the main theoretical points I would like to make here.

What can philosophy say about this case? Well, for one thing, if philosophy has really to do with *wisdom* as its etymology suggests, that is, with knowing-how to live well, it may help us to understand what went wrong in order to avoid similar cases happening again. It must, for instance, provide ways of making *wiser* decisions to avoid conflicts that increase suffering making in this way life better. This is not trivial since wisdom requires us to learn from our mistakes and escape repeating them. In order to achieve that, philosophy may use its critical powers to raise several other questions: (i) What are the values at stake, for instance, were the rights of Baby 1's parents really disrespected as the family's lawyer argued? (ii) Did caring require the health team to keep treating the patient or to let her die? (iii) Why did the parents first accept "*palliative*" *care* and then go to court to fight the decision to discontinue life support? (iv) Was *palliative care* conflated with passive euthanasia? (v) If any medical treatment was futile, why was active euthanasia not considered for the baby's own good? (vi) What were the roles of the media, the ethical committee and the legal system in this case? (vii) Why did the judge not give an immediate order to increase care? These are some general

[4] Hilde Lindemann, "Context: Backward, Sideways, and Forward" In: Rita Charon and Martha Montello (eds.) *Stories Matter,* (New York/London: Routledge, 2002), 40.

questions we need to answer in order to avoid similar cases happening again. Can a *philosophical* bioethics find a way of avoiding these cases? I believe so and I will try to show how throughout this book by proposing the concept of respectful care based on practical cognitivism.

It seems clear that, on the one hand, giving parents the last word may not be wise at all since they might desire what cannot be provided even by well-developed sciences and advanced technologies in very rich countries such as the US. That is why parents can have a say, but perhaps not the last word. Should doctors have it? I will in this work argue that this is not the case either. There is not yet a Carmentis Machine, that is, a device to ensure 100% certainty on diagnosis about, for instance, the kind of impairments Baby 1 would face if she could be saved.[5] On the other hand, the technological imperative must also be limited by philosophy: from an ethical point of view, it is not true that what *can* be done *must* always be. Technology, as applied science, is basically *knowing-how* to produce artefacts to transform our world. *How* to use them, however, whether to kill or to save lives, is a further and distinct issue, an ethical one. Perhaps the most important question philosophy of technology has to answer is this: how best to decide that what can be done need not be done? The case of Baby 1 shows us that not always what *can* be done (e.g., a transplantation of intestine) *ought* to be. Therefore, science and technology need wisdom to guide them. They need philosophy to show the way to a better life. They cannot be transformed into ends-in-themselves. More importantly, moral values cannot be driven by the needs of science and technology or by the religious convictions of any particular person. I will return this point in the last chapter.

I would now like to illustrate this point by taking into consideration, so to speak, the metaphysical battle behind the scenes in Baby 1's case. Briefly speaking, a health professional team must take a naturalist, a *scientific* stance towards the world, and the doctors were in fact obliged to take this route. That is to say, their religious beliefs must not interfere in their professions. On the other hand, the family and many commentators on the blog about this case, who were trying to influence the family's decisions, had a different worldview, a *religious*, even a fundamentalist one. To recognise that point, contrast what the parents of Baby 1 wrote in their posts, namely, "The clinical statistics for the 23 week old babies are not very good. But our faith is strong and we trust the Lord will see her thru," with this comment on their blog: "God is not the one who has kept

[5] For an explanation of how such a Carmentis Machine would work see: Dominic Wilkinson, *Death or Disability*? (Oxford: Oxford University Press, 2013), 5f. I will discuss Wilkinson's threshold framework for decision-making later.

this baby alive, MAN is. Babies born at that gestation do not live without aggressive medical intervention … and even with that, most die anyway. You cannot live without an intestine."

Now, philosophy is neither science nor religion and it must remain *agnostic* about metaphysical disputes. Thus, philosophy starts to help in this case in a particular way, namely by showing that much of the struggle around Baby 1 may just have been based on a mistaken contraposition between science and religion. The beginning of wisdom is to recognize the limits of human knowledge. In other words, philosophy sets *the limits* to both science and religion, clarifying their proper domains. Thus, a scientist cannot, for instance, expect miracles; a religious person may hope for a supernaturalist intervention in the causal chain of facts. But the relevant ethical question is this: what about Baby 1 *herself*? To be in the middle of a metaphysical dispute seems certainly detrimental to the patient. Philosophy can help to adjudicate this case by first of all showing that the metaphysical battle may be obfuscating what must be done for the sake of the baby's welfare. That is to say, metaphysical disputes are irresolvable and that means that either a theist or an atheist person (the parents or the medical team) must *care* in a proper way, for instance, by not doing more harm than benefit to the baby *herself*. She is the centre of respectful care. We may conclude, then, that such statements as "To someone to try to play God, it is not right," as Baby 1's mother said, have no role in deciding what to do in her case. They cannot, certainly, be taken seriously from an ethico-philosophical point of view. Consequently, in order to take a non-metaphysical stance towards a particular case, one must embrace *agnosticism* as a basic tenet for building up *a* common, sharable morality. It is a sign of wisdom to keep oneself out of metaphysical disputes, focusing instead on what the cared for's basic needs are.

I would now like to illustrate further how philosophy may help in similar cases by *critically* reflecting on the many moral issues involved. Philosophy's job is above all to put the relevant ethical questions on the table and not necessarily to try to answer them immediately. Now, the case of Baby 1 raises several interrogations about the underlying values, and some of these are *moral* ones: what were the intentions of the family in starting a blog? What kind of comment should be allowed on the internet (for instance, two comments accused doctors of condemning the baby to starvation), and is there a way of assessing them? Why did the parents *delete* some comments posted on their blog, were they trying to manipulate the public perception of the case? Do patients have a duty, not only a right, to confidentiality? What is the role of blogs in medicine, for example, can they be used to disclose information to patients? Should we create, in the name of transparency, a record of patients through publically accessible blogs? Could we ever think of a "public follow up system" for doctors and nurses anywhere to give their opinions on this and on similar cases?

Here are some more questions: what is the power-play role of the media in a case like this since the baby's family intentionally called a local TV channel after being instigated by comments on the blog? Were AA News and Channel X (not their real names) too sensationalist in reporting the case? Who manipulates whom: the media by "selecting" information or the public by "calling" the media when it is convenient to produce alarm or scandals? How can the media nowadays be more impartial and not surrender so easily to ideologies?

To continue questioning: what was the role of the legal system in this case? What kind of justice can be done by court order? Saving the baby's life or transplanting organs (intestines) even if it is pointless from a medical point of view? If the defendants requested a guardian *ad litem* to ensure the best interests of the child, what was left of the patient's autonomy in this case where she was legally represented by the parents? Were Baby 1's parents incompetent? Were the patient's rights completely violated, as the family's attorney argued in an interview for a TV channel? Did the court *disrespect* the baby herself by not giving an immediate order to increase *care*? Is this *fair* from a social, political point of view?

The questions do not stop there: what is the role of the (bio)ethics committee in this and similar cases? What kind of role may a paediatric ethics committee have? Must it have just an advisory and *educational* role or be part of the *decision-making* process also? In other words, must it have just a revisionary function or also the capacity to recommend a course of action? What about the composition of the ethics committee? Does it not represent corporate interests and protect the health professionals' interests given that the majority of its members come from the health institution itself? Is this composition of an ethics committee *ethical* after all?

What kind of principle (or value etc.) did the U. of A. apply to reach a conclusion about this particular case? Did it apply, for instance, the Hippocratic principle "first [or above all], *do no harm*?" as having an absolute status? If the answer is "yes" because any treatment is futile, that is, without therapeutic effect, would it not have been better *to euthanize* the baby instead of *withdrawing her food*?

There are other institutional questions: is a hospital entitled to refuse treatment if the parents have no proper health insurance (the patient was first transferred from another facility for insurance reasons and then denied a new transfer by the insurance company)? Is this fair from a *social* point of view? Should health caregivers withdraw treatment when it is futile without the patient's consent for economic reasons? If not, are they giving the appropriate, deserved care?

Consider also these questions: should they have given more treatment in the Baby 1 case, including more morphine (possibly hastening death), if the parents or the court had requested or demanded it? Were the doctors "playing God" (in the sense of deciding who should live or die), as the mother said in her interview with the TV channel? Would there have been a place for religion in this case if Baby 1 had happened to be in another facility? Were the parents and doctors rather disrespecting Nature by keeping Baby 1 alive by all means? Should the health team have tried an *experimental* transplantation, even if it is a risky and very expensive one, using the patient as an object (a mere means) of scientific research or have carried out a surgery to rip out parts of her intestine, which is also an invasive and perhaps unethical procedure, for teaching purposes only?

Certainly, there are other questions. If it is true, as the U. of A.'s unique short note on this case states, that "they met with the patient's parents and determined the most appropriate and ethically responsible course was palliative (end of life) care," why did the parents change their minds and go to court? How did the parents give the informed consent? Was it signed? Was clear information disclosed by the health team? Were the parents not entitled to change their minds and to demand the respect that the baby deserved, the care she really needed? Did they understand that palliative care *really* meant end of life care and, in this case, *withdrawing food*? It seems that the answer to this question was negative, as even the U. of A. defendant document recognizes, then, was this not a clearly disrespectful and uncaring attitude? And so on and so forth ...

I do not hope to answer all these questions in this book, but, as a philosopher and not as a professional bioethicist, I will certainly contribute to raising some more. My special concern is to ask whether what was absent was *respectful care* and how things could have turned out differently if Baby 1 had been cared for respectfully. Before trying to build up this concept, I would like to present in a more detailed way the idea of a philosophical bioethics and what we can expect from it in discussing the meta-ethical and normative bases of bioethics.

1.2 The idea of a philosophical bioethics

I would now like to say a few preliminary words about the conception of bioethics that I will use throughout this work. Simply put, I take bioethics to be part of ethics understood as a *philosophical* discipline, not a scientific or theological one. There is clear evidence that bioethics was born as a philosophical project. For instance, some have argued that bioethics is best understood in terms of the knowledge needed to use scientific knowledge. For one, van Potter, the American oncologist until recently believed to have coined the word 'bioethics,' held that we need *a new kind of wisdom*, namely "'the knowledge of how to use knowledge' for man's survival and for improvement in the quality of life."[6] Bioethics was conceived in an age when technoscience was not always used to provide a better life: the Cold War could have led to the destruction of humanity; industry was polluting the environment etc. Thus, the origin of bioethics was a response to the misuses of technology demanding more wisdom and not only more scientific knowledge. In the same spirit, Arne Naess proposed the word 'ecosophy,' calling for a *wiser* attitude towards nature as a whole.[7] The common assumption was the need felt for a new relation towards the environment and non-human animals to overcome the dichotomies and radicalisms introduced by modern sciences and their unwise technological applications. These misapplications were driven by a positivist or scientificist worldview. Science and technology can, as was tragically proved by the two world wars, be used to destroy humanity, if not life as a whole on this little blue planet. This is definitely not a sign of wisdom, and we are in no better position nowadays. We should not forget that these menaces are still hanging around, as Professor Stephen Hawking warned us recently, namely that the development of full artificial intelligence (AI) could spell the end of the human race. To avoid artificial intelligence destroying us, we need to enhance our wisdom, not only our scientific knowledge. I will return to this point in the last chapter.

It seems then a mistake to speak in terms of "biomedical ethics or bioethics" as if they were the same thing as some important bioethicists still do.[8] As we know today, the word 'bioethics' was used for the first time back in 1927 by Fritz Jahr, who stated the following principle:

---

[6] Rensselaer van Potter, *Bioethics*, (New Jersey: Prentice-Hall, 1971), 1.

[7] Naess is reported to have said: "What we need today is a tremendous expansion of ecological thinking in what I call ecosophy. *Sophy* comes from the Greek term *Sophia*, 'wisdom,' which relates to ethics, norms, rules, and practice. Ecosophy, or deep ecology, then, involves a shift from science to wisdom." *Apud* Bill Devall and George Sessions, "Deep Ecology" in: James Sterba, *Earth Ethics*, (New Jersey: Prentice Hall, 2000), 155.

[8] Unfortunately, this reductionist view is still widely held, for instance, by Beauchamp and Childress in their book *Principles of Biomedical Ethics* (Oxford: Oxford University Press, 2013), p.vii.

"Respect every living being on principle as an end in itself and treat it, if possible, as such."[9] I will comment on this principle later, in chapter 7. What we need to bear in mind, then, is that *special bioethics*, both clinical and academic, conceived as a practical discipline dealing with biomedical issues, came to be predominant leaving a more holist approach, based on wisdom and on a concern for life as a whole, aside. Thus, to avoid misunderstandings, I will use the expression 'holistic bioethics' to refer to Jahr's principle as well as Potter's project of a 'global bioethics'. I will reserve the expression 'global bioethics' to refer to bioethical issues in the international arena, for instance, whether informed consent is needed only in developed countries or also in other nations with no specific legislation requiring it. Thus, I will use the expression 'special bioethics' to refer to the moral issues surrounding human experimentation, for instance, in the biomedical sciences. Finally, I will use *philosophical bioethics* for an ethical discipline based on wisdom connecting all these dimensions, that is, special, global and holistic bioethical issues.

This is perhaps the right place to say something more about the origins of bioethics and why it began to be seen just as a deontology or a professional ethics for scientists, mainly in the life and medical sciences, instead of a concern for life as a whole based on wisdom. The main reason was the extraordinary advances in the past 40 years in areas such as the above referred to, namely neonatology. But stories like Baby 1's should make us rethink the foundations of special bioethics and discuss its basic principles, especially the role that individual autonomy, this "all-American value," has come to play nowadays. Since the publication of the *Belmont Report*, a US official document, which will be carefully examined in the next chapter, there has been widespread disagreement about the best formulation of the fundamental principles of special bioethics, namely *respect for persons*, *beneficence* and *justice*. These are, however, ethico-philosophical problems; not scientific ones.

Despite the fact that we may use the word 'ethics' as a synonym for 'morals' (the words are simply interchangeable), we need to establish a distinction between *studying* morality from a philosophical point of view and simply *moralizing*. Consequently, ethics is taken here as a theoretical discipline, as a philosophical reflection upon moral phenomena including bioethical issues such as whether active euthanasia in Baby 1's case was not a better option. We need, then, a clearer understanding of ethics to clarify the nature of bioethics itself.

[9] Fritz Jahr, "Bio-Ethics". In: Amir Muzur and Hans-Martin Sass (eds.), *Fritz Jahr and the Foundations of Global Bioethics*, (Berlin: Lit Verlag, 2012), 4.

Before presenting the main domains of ethics so defined, I would like to point out some differences between 'ethics' and 'morality'. As a philosophical discipline, ethics is based on wisdom, that is, on knowing-how to live well. Ethics is a philosophical and not a scientific enterprise, which starts with a distinction between facts and values and from the assumption that the latter cannot be justified only empirically. As the reconstruction of the Baby 1 story showed, we need to separate facts and values to better understand the particularities of the case in order to know what to do and, more importantly, *how* to do it. There may be sciences of moral phenomena, for instance, a sociological and statistical study of how many premature babies below 500gr do survive in a particular country (US or Brazil or UK), but bioethics is not among them. Ethics is about what we *must* or *must not do*, for instance, whether it is morally permissible to kill a chronically ill baby instead of let her die, and this is not an empirical question. That is to say, it does not depend on what is prescribed in a particular jurisdiction.

A moral system, on the other hand, may involve a set of habits, rules, qualities of character etc. of a group or society, which guide behaviour towards some conception of the good life. Consider Roger Crisp's characterization of a moral system:

> A set of cognitive and conative states, including beliefs, desires, and feelings, which leads its possessors among other things to (*a*) view certain actions as wrong (that is, morality forbidden) and hence to be avoided, (*b*) feel guilt and/or shame as a result of performing such actions, and (*c*) blame others who perform such actions.[10]

In this sense, as a matter of fact, there are many moral systems, many moralities: Jewish morality, Christian morality, socialist morality, Piraha's morality, Buddhist morality, Islamic morality, Hindu morality etc. etc. Whether there is a *common* morality is a further and distinct question. I will return to this point in chapter 4.

We must bear in mind, however, that ethics is *not* moral theology, that is, the application of a particular religious doctrine to the problems of life. It may be misleading, then, to assume from the very beginning that all these moral systems have their own particular bioethics. Of course, a specific religion may inform some bioethical issues such as whether euthanasia is permissible, but its beliefs and values cannot be universalized. Thus, pluralism has a limited role to play in a common morality. A principle such as "first, do no harm" may have an *a priori*

---

[10] Roger Crisp, *Reasons & the Good*, (Oxford: Oxford University Press, 2006), 9.

justification and, consequently, needs to be part of all moral systems enforcing a public web of norms. It is a philosophical task to discuss whether this is the case.

The word 'moral' may be used as a synonym for 'altruistic behaviour.' This is a predominant use in many scientific studies dealing with moral phenomena, such as psychology, ethnology etc. But this use excludes crucial moral concerns such as self-care and self-respect. Thus, I prefer to make a little modification here and use this sense of 'moral' as *intrinsically valuing someone*. In this work, I will also apply this use to characterize the moral value of caring & respecting as the main ingredients of *a* common, sharable morality.

In order then to achieve a better understanding of the nature of bioethical problems as belonging to the domain of ethics as a philosophical discipline, I will now specify in a more detailed way each of its subareas. Ethics is composed of three domains: *meta-ethics*, *normative ethics* and *applied ethics*, and bioethics is a subdomain of applied or practical ethics. Now, *meta-ethics* deals with the form, the structure and the nature of ethics itself. Meta-ethics is a philosophical reflection on the logical, ontological and epistemic status of ethics. It is not something above or beyond ethics, but it is part of its own self-questioning. For instance, it is a meta-ethical question whether ethics might be considered a science among others. That is to say, whether ethics may take the form of a theory or whether it should rely on principles or moral qualities such as virtues etc. It is worth pointing out here that bioethics was originally conceived as a project for re-unifying ethical *values* and biological *facts*, and that is a metabioethical question which is still much discussed.[11] Bioethics itself was designed to bridge the *is-ought gap* between how the world *is* (sciences) and how we *ought* to behave (humanities), the so called "two cultures," and to build a new science of our survival. In presenting the case of Baby 1, I took a different path: I have tried to *distinguish* facts from values. This was a meta-ethical decision. Now, the other meta-ethical questions are: what do the moral words 'good,' 'right,' 'duty,' 'care,' 'respect' etc. mean? Is there a moral primitive concept from which the others can be defined, if so, which is the moral primitive term 'good' or 'right'? If it is 'good,' then does it follow necessarily a teleological or consequentialist normative ethical approach? If it is 'right,' then does it imply a deontological one? Can we use a non-priority thesis between 'good' and 'right' to integrate

[11] Rensselaer van Potter, *Bioethics*, (New Jersey: Prentice-Hall, 1971), p. vii. However, as I have argued in the past years (2000, 2013c), to conflate facts and values is to commit the naturalistic fallacy, which I take basically to be a category mistake. We must, so to speak, avoid criss-crossing language games.

caring & respecting, defining them in terms of intrinsic value? What is the nature of moral judgments? Are moral judgments objective and, if so, in what sense? Can moral judgments be true or false? In what sense? Is there moral knowledge as cognitivist meta-ethicists hold? Are there moral facts that can warrant such objectivity? Which is the best method in bioethics? And so on. In presenting practical cognitivism in chapter 5 to replace the intuitionist meta-ethics of the predominant normative bioethical theory, I will answer most of these questions.

Somehow interconnected with meta-ethical issues, *normative ethics* deals with ways of positively establishing the distinction between good and bad, right and wrong etc. It may work with principles, procedures, values, rights, or any other criterion to make such a discrimination between what is morally obligatory, permissible or forbidden. The three main approaches to normative ethics nowadays are *virtue ethics*, *deontology* and *consequentialism*. They inform also the bioethical debates represented, for instance, by the works of Edmund Pellegrino, Tristram Engelhardt and Tom Beauchamp, a virtue ethicist, a deontologist and a utilitarian, respectively. I will discuss their works in the next two chapters. Roughly speaking, *virtue ethics* holds that the good person, the good character, that is, the person who has moral qualities is the model to be followed and that an action is right if and only if it is the one the virtuous agent would perform in the circumstances. *Deontological* theories hold that there is a principle such as the Golden Rule (one should treat others as one would like others to treat oneself), or a set of principles or procedures, which establish what is the right and obligatory action, independently of the results or an appeal to the good. Finally, *consequentialism* is the view that holds the best outcome as the criterion to be taken into consideration when deliberating whether or not an action must be performed. A more detailed explanation of these theories will be given throughout this book. In chapter 5, I will propose a way of integrating these three normative approaches by amending Derek Parfit's Triple Theory.

The referred to predominant view in special bioethics is, normatively speaking, a "mixed" theory. That is to say, principlism tries to combine norms which are deontological (e.g., respect for autonomy or justice) with consequentialist-oriented ones (for instance, beneficence). Furthermore, this account is meta-ethically speaking *intuitionist* in Rawls' sense, namely it assumes that there is no single, fundamental principle of morality like the classical modern philosophers Immanuel Kant and John Stuart Mill and, more recently, Derek Parfit held. An intuitionist also denies that we can *rank* moral principles giving priority to, let us say, individual autonomy over beneficence. This may bring additional problems since a moral dilemma as it appeared in the case of Baby 1, a conflict in the application of either the principle of respect for parents' autonomy or a beneficent course of action in the patient's best interests, can lead to inaction if there is no way of solving it. Thus, in this book, when I speak of "re-thinking the meta-ethical basis of bioethics" the main point I am referring to is whether the intuitionist basis of principlism is sustainable given that it leads to such moral dilemmas. Moreover, it seems a common practice, especially in most North-American textbooks on bioethics (also in Law), to start by spelling out the main ethical theories, for example, consequentialism, deontology, virtue ethics, feminist ethics etc. as well as the rejection of theories put forward, for instance, by casuistry, without providing any clue about how to overcome this very confusing "state of art." This phenomenon is sometimes called "the textbook approach." It leads straightaway to relativism, if not to moral scepticism. Thus, another meta-ethical issue I would like to discuss is whether relativism is a consequence of the intuitionist basis of bioethics. Some positive proposals to overcome this state of affairs such as Engelhardt's autonomism and Pellegrino's beneficence-in-trust model will be discussed in this context. Finally, one of the main challenges in normative bioethics nowadays is to find a way of integrating *prima facie* principles, perhaps using a metaprinciple. The main concept presented here aims to overcome this problem by combining care & respect into a fundamental attitude. How this can be done will become apparent later.

Practical ethics is the application of normative accounts to particular cases taking into consideration the results of meta-ethical and normative investigations. Now, bioethics is a special branch of applied ethics as are environmental ethics, animal ethics, information ethics, machine ethics, professional ethics (for physicians, journalists, lawyers, paediatricians, nurses etc.) and so on. Now, as we have seen, despite the fact that bioethics was meant to include ethical considerations on the environment and non-human animals in van Potter's work (what he called 'global ethics'), nowadays it is predominantly confined to *academic* special bioethics (mainly in scientific research) and *clinical* special bioethics. Kinds of bioethics may, however, be distinguished but not separated since a physician may have a dual role – as a researcher and as a doctor treating a patient – yet there are clear connections here. Thus, I will restrict myself to *special bioethics* in the next five chapters, but this does not mean that I am doing *medical* ethics. I will deal with some global and holistic bioethical issues in the last chapter. Now, neonatal bioethics is a branch of special bioethics. It is also important to clarify that restricting special bioethics to research involving human subjects does not imply that I am assuming an anthropocentric stance.

The integration of special, global and holistic bioethics is made by the idea of a philosophical bioethics. A bioethical study is philosophical when it uses speculative methods (not experimental ones), which are interrogative, critical and argumentative, and try to understand the world as a whole. In this sense, it is distinct from a scientific study, let me say, ethnological or sociological about, for instance, abortion or euthanasia in a particular group or society, which would use observation, empirical data, analysis of variables, hypotheses, etc. and in the end construct a theory to explain a particular moral phenomenon with no normative implications. Ethics, as a philosophical discipline, must be capable of understanding normativity in its specific properties. For instance, it needs to present a justification for judgments such as: doctors *must* withhold futile treatment and let the patient die.

This book tries as far as possible to combine the three dimensions of ethical inquiry: meta-ethical, normative and applied. This is another meaning of what I called 'philosophical bioethics', that is, a reflection on moral issues of life and death guided by wisdom. To illustrate, I will conduct a metabioethical analysis of 'care' and 'respect' in chapter 4 *and* find out their normative implications in order to apply them to particular neonatal moral problems. Despite the fact that the relationships between meta-ethical theories and normative approaches are not always clear, there is a connection between them. For instance, a consequentialist normative ethics most of the time goes with realism. Now, meta-ethics has priority from a philosophical point of view, but there is no doubt that concrete bioethical issues have more urgency from a daily perspective. Throughout this work, I will construct from a philosophical perspective the concept of respectful care referring to an attitude capable of dealing with practical issues including bioethical problems.

Before finishing this section, I would like to recall Baby 1's story in order to show that real wisdom was absent despite all the technological and scientific developments, and that this was one of the problems concerning the case. Lantos and Meadow are after all right: doctors didn't *know-how* to apply the Baby Doe guidelines and some still do not know. Now, it is not only true that "the founding fathers" (Fritz Jahr and van Potter) of bioethics were pushing for more wisdom, nothing else, but also that some bioethicists still continue in their tradition. Against Johnston's disbelief in wisdom and his defence of bioethics as "the mastery of a technique,"[12] I believe that we need more wisdom, not more expertise. To provide an example from our story: it was not *a wise decision* to let Baby 1 die telling the parents that palliative care would be provided, without explaining in very clear language what the health team would in fact do, that is, withdraw vital support.

What else can philosophy, conceived as pursuit of wisdom, do for bioethics? To answer this question, let me recall another source of the origin of bioethics as a *special* discipline somehow related to biomedical studies only. As Daniel Callahan, the director of the Hastings Center, an institution that played a major role in making bioethics what it is today together with the Kennedy Institute, points out in his famous 1973 paper "Bioethics as a Discipline," philosophers can help physicians and biologists. How? Well-trained ethicists can: "analyze concepts, clarify principles, see logical entailments, spot underlying assumptions, and build theoretical systems."[13] These are certainly not easy tasks. Albert Jonsen also holds that philosophers came into bioethics by working on "clarifying the concepts".[14] As I have already pointed out, I will try above all in this work to analyse the concept *respectful care*. This concept has been neglected by many bioethicists and health professionals alike. It seems that it could have prevented many cases such as Baby 1's story. Respectful care is paramount in guiding our moral lives. Thus, one methodological strategy that I will follow in this work is analysing, in the rather narrow sense of 'analysis,' the concepts central to bioethics, namely care & respect, to see whether they match. Once I have done that, we can redefine these concepts and then examine the conditions for a respectful caring attitude.

There are, however, more things philosophers can do. According to Callahan, methodological investigations are not the only contribution that philosophers can bring to bioethics; building up theoretical systems is also a task for them. I am engaging in such an enterprise here when discussing what is *a common, sharable morality* from an ethico-philosophical perspective. I will argue that such a system is capable of adjudicating the conflicts at stake in Baby 1's case. Again, all we need is more wisdom.

We may then conclude that wisdom is crucial in bioethics just as it is elsewhere. Consider how disastrous the outcome of the Baby 1 case was.

---

[12] Paul Johnston, "Bioethics, Wisdom, and Expertise." In: Carl Elliot (ed.), *Show Cures, Bad Philosophers*, (Durham/London: Duke University Press, 2001), 157.

[13] Daniel Callahan, "Bioethics as a Discipline." In: Nancy Jecker *et al.* (eds) *Bioethics* (Sudbury: Jones and Bartlett, 2007), 19.

[14] Albert R. Jonsen, *The Birth of Bioethics*, (New York/Oxford: Oxford University Pres, 1998), 65.

There was the suspicion of negligence, if not malpractice; a breakdown in communication between the health team and the family happened at some point; the ethics committee did not make a wise decision to avoid a litigation process; the judicial system did not help etc. etc. and … the baby died. We do need *wiser* health professionals, *wiser* hospital administrators, *wiser* judges, *wiser* parents, *wiser* journalists etc. It is a sad reality, but bioethics is failing to contribute to a *wiser* society and, consequently, to a better world. It is time to start to reverse this state of affairs by engaging ourselves in a more *philosophical* bioethics.

CHAPTER TWO

RETHINKING THE META-ETHICAL BASIS OF SPECIAL BIOETHICS

Despite the fact that the predominant normative approach in special bioethics is a principled one based on the *prima facie* norms of respect for autonomy, non-maleficence, beneficence and justice, many philosophers believe that this is the wrong methodological strategy. The reason is simple: there are no *universal* principles, they argue. All casuists, some feminists, most virtue ethicists etc. hold that there are no universal norms or, if they exist, they would be too formal to be useful in deciding what to do in particular cases. All these methodological trends have in common a *particularist* approach to moral problems. Others argue, however, that almost any principle can be universalized, but which one must be applied in particular cases is open to question, and that leads to fundamental disagreements, to dilemmas and ultimately to inaction. Thus, in the first section of this chapter, I will discuss some bioethical views which hold that there are no universal moral principles. In this sense, the referred to principles would be *general* guidelines only. This is an important issue related to whether we should use a methodology based on universal principles or instead on particular cases only. It is a meta-bioethical problem. I have introduced a particular case in chapter 1 and mentioned some *prima facie* principles based on the Belmont Report, which I will start to discuss in more detail in the second part of this chapter, scrutinizing its intuitionist meta-ethics.

2.1 Methodology: cases or principles?

Arguably, one of the most important developments in the field of special bioethics was the publication of the Belmont Report, in 1978. This document was the result of the workings of the National Commission for the Protection of Human Subjects of Bioemedical and Behavioral Research (from 1974 to 1978), in the US, and it came to be seen as a kind of constitution for bioethics sorting out three *prima facie* principles that must be used to assess the morality of scientific research involving human beings, the already referred to norms of respect for persons, beneficence and justice. In this section, I will start to discuss its significance and the many ethical questions it raised, especially methodological ones.

I would like to begin by pointing out that the Belmont Report is a special document in many senses. First, it was a response to the famous Tuskegee case, where persons were manipulated as mere objects of scientific research. Second, the Belmont Report seems to be a *compromise* (perhaps, in the pejorative, political sense) between ethicists of many different philosophical backgrounds. For instance, Tom Beauchamp, who was hired by the National Commission to write it, has a special interpretation of the nature of the principles, namely that the three basic norms are *universal*. Beauchamp is a utilitarianist in normative ethics, according to whom we must do the most good we can and only the consequences of our actions matter in establishing it. Other philosophers, who also worked as staff members for the commission, disagree. For someone defending a casuistic point of view, like the only philosopher working in the National Commission, namely Albert Jonsen, what could it mean to accept *prima facie* principles if not *generalizations* only? As the Wittgensteinian philosopher Stephen Toulmin, who worked as a consultant for the National Commission, wrote: "I was struck by the extent to which the commissioners were able to reach agreement in making recommendations about ethical issues of great complexity and delicacy."[1] Issues involving prisoners, mental patients and human foetuses were discussed and the recommendations were made with only residual differences in opinion; some "more conservative," others "more liberal". Puzzlingly enough, however, we now know that there was no theoretical consensus in the National Commission, although a practical accord was achieved. Thus, according to Jonsen and Toulmin, "Members of the commission were largely in agreement about their specific practical recommendations; they agreed what it was they agreed about; but the one thing they could not agree on was *why* they agreed about it."[2] Obviously, the casuists Jonsen and Toulmin thought that the Commission was not overly concerned with *universal* principles, but with *general* judgments about specific kinds of cases only.

---

[1] Stephen Toulmin, "How Medicine Saved the Life of Ethics." In: Nancy Jecker *et al.* (eds), *Bioethics*, (Sudbury: Jones and Bartlett Publishers, 2007), 27-28.

[2] Albert R. Jonsen and Stephen Toulmin, *The Abuse of Casuistry*, (Berkeley: University of California Press, 1988), 18.

This is a metabioethical point worth examining deeper. According to Toulmin, the problems arose not on what to do in particular cases, but at the justificatory level. He later asked himself:

> How was the Commission's consensus possible? It rested precisely on this last feature of their agenda namely, its close concentration of specific types of problematic cases. Faced with 'hard cases,' they inquired what particular conflicts of claim or interest were exemplified in them, and they usually ended by balancing off those claims in very similar ways. Only when the individual members of the Commission went on to explain their own particular 'reason' for supporting the general consensus did they begin to go seriously different ways. For, then, commissioners from different backgrounds and faiths 'justified' their votes by appealing to general views and abstract principles which differed far more deeply than their opinions about particular substantive questions. Instead of 'deducing' their opinions about particular cases from general principles that could lend strength and conviction to those specific opinions, they showed a far greater certitude about particular cases than they ever achieved about general matters.[3]

Stephen Toulmin, who co-authored the book *The Abuse of Casuistry* with the commissioner-philosopher Albert Jonsen, then, argued that the work of the Commission is a good illustration of applying the method of casuistry. I just wonder what they would recommend in a case such as Baby 1's: keep her alive indefinitely? Withdraw food? Take her life in a different manner? I am not sure casuists would agree on this particular case.

I would now like to focus on this methodological issue: after all, should we work with *cases* only or with *universal* principles instead? Should we use a "top-down" (from universal principles to cases) method of moral reasoning or rather some kind of "bottom-up" (from cases to general norms) model as represented by casuistry? To start to answer these questions, I would like to point out that I have so far followed many casuistic recommendations in presenting Baby 1: using real cases rather than hypothetical ones; avoiding schematic presentations etc. This, however, does not mean that I am necessarily sceptical regarding the existence of universal principles.

To be sure, casuistry prescribes that we have to:

i) pay attention to the morally relevant features of the case;
ii) find analogous cases or paradigms that share those features; and

---

[3] Stephen Toulmin, "How Medicine Saved the Life of Ethics." In: Nancy Jecker *et al* (eds), *Bioethics*, (Sudbury: Jones and Bartlett Publishers, 2007), 28.

iii) consider the maxim associated with the paradigm and use it to shed light on the case at hand.[4]

I also followed some of these recommendations in my analysis of the Baby 1 story, and I will use them again in presenting new bioethical cases. But casuistry holds that we should reject or modify a general ethical principle since there are no *universal* principles. This I find difficult to accept.

The best defence of casuistry in bioethics was really made by Jonsen and Toulmin out of their experience in the National Commission. They argued that the Commission worked “from the bottom,” that is, from the resolution of particular cases to the elaboration of the general principles as they now appear in the Belmont Report. Casuistry starts from the idea that moral knowledge is particular to circumstances, times and places. On the other hand, Beauchamp and Childress argued that the Commission is an example of the principled method, that is, “from the top”: we must apply universal principles to solve particular bioethical cases. Who is right, in the end? Jonsen and Toulmin’s book *The Abuse of Casuistry* argues for the primacy of moral cases over moral theory and principles. They hold that casuistry can achieve agreement across theoretical divides, thus providing moral foundations for bioethics. They have a particular understanding of casuistry: starting from cases, we should search for paradigmatic examples to establish what must be done, for instance, in Baby 1’s case. A problem for this methodology is this: should we use the Baby Doe case as the paradigmatic one to decide what to do with Baby 1 or another case instead? If we use the Baby Doe case, she should have been allowed to die, but her parents did not want that outcome. Thus, casuistry seems an incomplete method.

Many bioethicists have criticized the casuistic approach for denying that there are universal principles and for relying on different criteria for moral action. For instance, Kevin W. Wildes argues against Jonsen and Toulmin maintaining that the model of casuistry they deploy relies on moral authority for case interpretation (e.g., bishops) and, consequently, that they cannot succeed in a secular context that is morally pluralistic and, consequently, directed by different moral views. This is in fact a crucial point since special bioethics must consider the fact of pluralism.[5] Wildes

---

[4] Nancy Jecker “Methods of Ethical Reasoning: Philosophical, Clinical, and Cultural Dimensions.” In: Nancy Jecker *et al.* (eds), *Bioethics*, (Sudbury: Jones and Bartlett Publishers, 2007), 105.

[5] This can be recognized in the composition of the National Commission itself: “The eleven commissioners had varied backgrounds and interests. They included men and women; blacks and whites; Catholics, Protestants, Jews, and atheists;

concludes then that "like the ancient world and the confessional practices of the early Middle Ages, there is a plurality of casuistries in the contemporary world."[6] Again, a Catholic bioethicist such as Albert Jonsen himself, if he follows the official doctrine, would not support withdrawing food in the Baby 1 case. I will return to this point in chapter 4 while discussing whether we should kill or let die patients in such conditions from the point of view of *a* common, sharable morality. Another bioethicist, perhaps a Protestant one or an atheist, could decide differently. Therefore, the success of the National Commission was due to "shared moral intuitions" or because its members were "moral acquaintances," that is, they were among friends.

At this juncture, it is worth underlining the fact that bioethical methods are distinct from scientific ones. Consider how medicine, particularly neonatology, is based on many natural sciences, for instance, on the basic biological facts of human anatomy such as the intestines' role in keeping someone alive by providing nutrients. Moreover, evidence-based medicine may even use statistics, for instance, in order to show that an ELBW baby with 23 weeks of gestation has <10% survival rate, a 15/25% chance of being severely disabled etc.[7] Medicine, however, is a complex kind of *art*: it may use the natural sciences, even exact ones such as mathematics, but it always has a *singular individual*, a particular patient, to heal and this brings additional methodological problems. For example, recent developments in neuroscience and neuroethics may help neonatologists to check whether an extremely premature baby has suffered severe brain damage. They cannot, however, set a bioethical question such as whether we should euthanize the patient or just let her die. The central *ethico-philosophical* question is what we *must* do and this is a *normative* issue, not a *descriptive* one. One may perhaps grasp the specificities in a very simple example: to describe "withdrawing mechanical ventilation kills the baby" is not to prescribe "the ventilation *must* be withdrawn". These

---

medical scientists and behaviorist psychologists; philosophers; lawyers; theologians; and public interest representatives." Albert R. Jonsen and Stephen Toulmin, *The Abuse of Casuistry*, (Berkeley: University of California Press, 1988), 17. See also Tom Beauchamp "The Origins and Evolution of the Belmont Report" in: James F. Childress *et al.* (eds.), *Belmont Revisited*, (Washington: Georgetown University Press, 2005), 12f.

[6] Kevin, Wildes, *Moral Acquaintances*, (Notre Dame: University of Notre Dame Press, 2000), 120.

[7] Norman Campbell "When Care Cannot Cure: Medical Problems in Seriously Ill Babies." In: Helga Kuhse and Peter Singer (eds), *Bioethics*, (Oxford: Blackwell, 2006), 307.

statements are different in *kind,* as are science and philosophical bioethics. They are composed of, so to speak, different language-games. I will return to this Wittgensteinian idea in chapter 5.

For the question "cases or principles?" there is no easy way out, but it can perhaps be answered in a non-dogmatic way. Thus, I will simply start by supposing that there may be universal moral principles and ask particularists to offer a counter-example rejecting them. In order to avoid dogmatism, this is perhaps the best place then to present a clear illustration of a top-down, deductivist, way of practical reasoning. It can be done using the previous case:

P1 (Major Premise): all persons are morally forbidden to produce more harms than benefits;
P2 (Minor Premise): performing an intestine transplantation on Baby 1 produces more harm than good;
Conclusion: the health team must not perform it.

We can dispute whether P2 is true, but I do not see any exemption to the principle that we must bring about more benefits than harms. As we will see in chapter 5, denying P1 makes morality unintelligible for our lifeform.

Bioethicists defending a deductivist approach start by sorting out basic principles such as respect for persons or non-maleficence etc., which are considered universal, and seek the application of such primitive norms in a deductive way to particular cases. To deny that there are such universal principles becomes, consequently, an *onus probandi* for the particularists since it seems simply self-evident that one does not act rightly by causing more harms than benefits. It does not follow that a deductivist bioethicist must be insensitive to or neglect the singularities of particular cases.

One could, in fact, object that principles such as P1 are too general, empty, abstract, formal; that even *specificication* (sorting out particular rules such as "do not kill innocent people" from universal principles like non-maleficence), a remedy developed by principlists to avoid these difficulties, is not sufficient and that therefore casuistry is the best way around. Moreover, one could hold, supposedly based on Wittgenstein's later philosophy, that principles cannot guide action effectively. For example, Jamie Nelson argued that there is an "in-principle-uneliminable ambiguity of rules".[8] For this reason, he presented an alternative approach,

8 James Lindemann Nelson "'Unlike Calculating Rules'? Clinical Judgement, Formalized Decision Making, and Wittgenstein." In: Carl Elliot (ed.), *Show Cures and Bad Philosophers*, (Durham/London: Duke University Press, 2001), 60.

the so-called "expert judgment model," which does not see principles as algorithms for any kind of circumstance and relies on *phronesis* (practical wisdom) instead. Granted, a "formal evidence model" purely based on statistics would perhaps be rejected by Wittgenstein, but Nelson's scepticism relies on a misleading reading of the rule-following considerations. I will return to this point in chapter 5. Moreover, Jamie Nelson has not shown that Wittgenstein would not be concerned with describing the facts and values of our human lifeform (*Lebensform*). If this is right, then Toulmin's communitarian reading of this concept is wrong too.[9] Besides, Wittgenstein explicitly wrote: "There is something universal here; not just something personal."[10] Examples in bioethics may include the above P1. Therefore, Wittgenstein is not a sufficient authority for denying that there are universal moral principles. Moreover, Nelson's "expert judgment model" may, even if it were right, be committed to paternalist assumptions, and it does not preclude the need for informed consent, that is, effective engagement with a patient's desires, preferences etc.

The same criticism seems to apply to *narrative* approaches in bioethics. According to Hilde Lindemann, who works with narrative ethics, "moral principles are not lawlike, universal, and unyielding, but modifiable in light of the particulars of a given experience or situation" and "these particulars either naturally take a narrative form or must be given a narrative structure if they are to have moral meaning."[11] Thus, a fundamental philosophical question is whether stories are sufficient to guide what to do. It seems, however, that John Arras is right when he argues that stories can only be a *supplement* to a principlist ethics, but not

---

Despite the fact that I agree with Jamie Nelson on the importance of *phronesis* in our moral lives, I do not believe that we can make a particularist reading of the Aristotelian ethics either.

[9] Toulmin wrote: "We find ourselves born into communities in which the available ways of acting are largely laid out in advance: in which human activity takes on different *Lebensformen,* or 'forms of life' (of which the professions are one special case), and our obligations are shaped by the requirements of those forms." Stephen Toulmin, "How Medicine Saved the Life of Ethics." In: Nancy Jecker *et al* (eds), *Bioethics*, (Sudbury: Jones and Bartlett Publishers, 2007), 30. I will return to the concept of 'lifeform' in chapter 5 providing a different interpretation.

[10] Ludwig Wittgenstein, *On Certainty*, §440.

[11] Hilde Lindemann Nelson, *Stories and Their Limits*, (New York: Routledge, 1997), p.ix.

the very ground for moral *justification*.[12] No one can deny that stories like Baby 1's may be told in order to learn something from them. I have learned a lot and I hope the reader will too. But it is also clear that stories are good tools for *moral education*, for moral learning only. For instance, one lesson that a health professional team can pick up from the Baby 1 story is that *communication* is paramount not only between doctors and patients (or their parents), but among the obstetrician and paediatrician, the social workers, the nurses etc. themselves. This certainly holds the potential to avoid subsequent problems. A layperson may learn that what she prefers in terms of treatment cannot always be done: no one can buy a new small intestine for Baby 1, and thus that the principle "above all, do no harm," which is a common sense principle after all, should be followed also by common people and not just by doctors out of their Hippocratic oath. But stories have little to say about *moral justification*. A principle such as the Hippocratic Imperative is self-evident because pain and suffering are just bad in themselves. There is no need to present further reasons. Thus, a principle forbidding doing more harms than benefits seems even to have an *a priori* justification. To use a Wittgensteinian jargon, which will be clarified in chapter 5, it is a *hinge*-proposition to say that it is wrong to cause more harms than good. This seems true in the Baby 1 case as it is in any other. Even with Baby Doe, who according to *some* casuists may be used as the paradigmatic case for deciding what to do in the Baby 1 story, the course of action was perhaps decided taking into consideration the universality of the non-maleficence principle. I will return to this point when discussing the norm of non-maleficence in a more detailed way in chapter 4.

Many authors, even particularist ones, concede that we can issue moral judgments that travel well beyond individual cases, but "… there *are* no rules or principles, even enormously complicated ones, capable of codifying the moral landscape."[13] But perhaps there are universal moral principles and also universal requirements to apply them. A principle such

[12] John Arras, "Nice Story, But so What? Narrative and Justification in Ethics." In: Jecker, Nancy *et al* (eds). *Bioethics*. (Sudbury: Jones and Bartlett Publishers, 2007), 212.

[13] Margaret Olivia Little has also argued in "Lessons on Moral Particularism" for a non-universalist ethics supposedly from a Wittgensteinian perspective (p.162f). But she seems to make the same mistaken interpretation of Wittgenstein's rule-following considerations failing to recognize that between Rule-Platonism and Rule-skepticism, there is a better alternative. I will, in chapter 5, propose a better reading of the rule-following considerations, but Magie Little is right in holding that the moral life cannot be *reduced* to rules.

as "for all persons, it is necessary not to cause more harms than benefits" seems to be a universal norm, which must be applied taking into consideration the particularities of the case, the contexts etc., but cannot be subverted. I can imagine no counterexample to this principle.

Now, the word 'universality' may even have different meanings. As Richard Hare argued in different works, similar cases must be judged similarly. This is the idea of universalizability, not that a principle holds for *all* agents in *all* circumstances. It is certainly a sound basis for a fair judgment and it is another universal principle that even casuists must accept while considering justice. It is not only inconsistent to deny that we must judge similar cases equally; it is immoral. That is to say, similar cases must be judged similarly. For instance, if any other ELBW baby had NEC in similar circumstances, the same decision with respect to non-maleficence must be taken. Thus, since stories and isolated cases cannot help in deciding what to do, one should instead ask what the justified principles are and apply them correctly. Philosophy can, therefore, help bioethics to find the best approach to its problems.

Another thing that philosophy can do is help special bioethics out of the current methodological maze. Here is then my suggestion regarding the question "cases or principles?": let us consider moral reasoning in terms of the Aristotelian notion of practical syllogisms as a prudent person, that is, what someone with practical wisdom (*phronesis*), would deliberate in deciding what to do. I provided an example above. The major premise can be taken as a universal principle (for instance, non-maleficence); the minor premise, as a particular judgment stating whether a case falls under the first premise (e.g., whether transplanting Baby 1's intestine produces more harms than benefits) and the conclusion, a prescription about what to do in a particular case in order to follow the universal norm. If this is the right account of practical reasoning, then one may recognize that principles without cases are empty and that cases without universal principles are blind. We need both in our practical deliberations.

It is a different matter to ask: *what* are these principles? In the next section, I will start to answer that question by reconstructing the main principles of the Belmont Report in a more detailed way and then discussing some proposals to complement or rectify this bioethical framework. The addition of new principles, which was somehow foreseen by the Belmont Report itself, is nowadays very common and must be taken into account while re-thinking the meta-ethical and normative bases of bioethics.

2.2 The Belmont's intuitionist framework

As we have seen in the last section, the Belmont Report was a special bioethical document establishing the main ethical framework for bioethics based on the principles of respect for persons, beneficence and justice. As we will now see, however, some bioethicists (e.g., Miller) argued that it must be complemented by different norms, for instance, by the principle of the sanctity of life; others (e.g., Beauchamp) maintained that respect for *autonomy* and not respect for *persons* is required; others held that we must rank one of these principles, namely either autonomy (e.g., Engelhardt) or beneficence (e.g., Pellegrino) over the others. I will discuss all these *normative* bioethical approaches in this and in the next chapter, but as I said in the introduction, the main purpose of this book is to call for a change in attitude, a call for a respectful caring manner in special bioethics. Thus, despite the fact that one should not reduce the moral life to norms and rules, a preliminary discussion of the fundamental bioethical norms established by the Belmont Report is paramount in understanding a respectful caring manner of acting. The reason is that an attitude requires the internalization of norms, both principles and rules.

To start with, it is worth pointing out that the National Commission had the following task: "identify the ethical *principles* which should underlie the conduct of biomedical and behavioural research with human subjects and develop guidelines that should be followed in such research" (italics added).[14] To some extent, it was very successful in accomplishing this particular task. The document relied on previous international texts such as The Nuremberg Code and The Declaration of Helsinki. It is worth pointing out that The Nuremberg Code was the first document to establish the need for informed consent in scientific research involving humans. Now, Commissioner Albert Jonsen, the only philosopher who was an effective member of the National Commission, recalls in his book *The Birth of Bioethics* the way they arrived at just three principles and nothing else. According to Jonsen, Commissioner Lebacqz delivered the work of the ethical-principles group selecting the following basic norms: respect; self-determination; benefit for individual research subjects; benefit for other individuals and groups present and future; minimization of harms to individual subjects; minimization of consequential harms to others and attendance to distributive justice and to compensating justice.[15] Some

[14] See: Albert R. Jonsen, *The Birth of Bioethics*, (Oxford: Oxford University Press, 1998), 102.

[15] Albert R. Jonsen, *The Birth of Bioethics*, (Oxford: Oxford University Press, 1998), 103.

commissioners complained that there were too many principles, that some were not universal and called for "crisp" fundamental norms. Jonsen then reveals that after much discussion, the commissioners took Engelhardt's first two principles [respect for persons as free moral agents; concern to support the best interests of human subjects in research, intent in assuring that the use of human subjects in experimentation will on the sum redound to the benefit of society] and Beauchamp's principle of distributive justice, and crafted "crisp" principles: *respect for persons, beneficence* and *justice*.

Who wrote the final version of the Belmont Report, however, is still disputed nowadays. Stephen Toulmin argued that he redrafted a report in March 1976, which came to be known as *The Belmont Report*, but Tom Beauchamp, who was specially appointed to write the document, thinks that he produced the final version, while Albert Jonsen said that it was in his home in San Francisco that the final document was written.[16] Leaving this "paternity" issue aside here, let me scrutinize each principle of the Belmont Report since it is the basis for other approaches such as classical principlism and to some extent autonomism and beneficence-in-trust, which will be discussed in the next chapter.

One of the fundamental *prima facie* principles of the Belmont Report is this:

a) Respect for Persons

The document explicitly recommends as an action-guiding norm respect for *persons*, not just autonomy. This principle received the following formulation:

> Respect for persons incorporates at least two ethical convictions: first, that individuals should be treated as autonomous agents, and second, that persons with diminished autonomy are entitled to protection. The principle of respect for persons thus divides into two separate moral requirements: the requirement to acknowledge autonomy and the requirement to protect those with diminished autonomy.

Many bioethicists understand this principle as requiring more than just respect for autonomous decisions or choices since it also states that persons with diminished autonomy are entitled to protection. Recalling our

---

[16] I will refer to this document as it appears in James F. Childress *et al.* (eds), *Belmont Revisited. Ethical Principles for Research with Human Subjects*, (Washington: Georgetown University Press, 2005), p.253-265. See also an online version at: http://www.hhs.gov/ohrp/humansubjects/guidance/belmont.html

bioethical case, Baby 1 is certainly protected under the principle of respect for persons, but it is unclear whether she would be under a principle of respect just for autonomy since she is unable to deliberate, to choose and to decide what to do. There is, obviously, the figure of the surrogate or substituted judgement, but the Belmont Report is particularly careful when it states that respect for the immature and the incapacitated may require protecting them as they mature or while they are disabled. One of the main problems with the principle of respect for autonomy, in the sense of individual self-determination, is that it may be subjected to a physician's judgment whether an individual lacks autonomy or not. Thus, the power seems to remain within the medical team to determine this, just as it was in the Hippocratic tradition. If a patient disagrees with a doctor's diagnostics or prognostics, she could ask for a psychological assessment. This may become a dark side of the doctor's power indeed.

The occurrence of the word 'person' in the Belmont Report, however, should not necessarily be considered a sign that a metaphysical assumption was in place. Downie and Telfer's book, namely *Respect for Persons,* which influenced the formulation of this principle, establishes two conditions for an individual to be considered a person*:* the capacity for self-determination and rule-following.[17] Perhaps, the latter includes the former. In fact, this is the sense that I will adopt for 'person' throughout this work: *a rule-following being*. This is neither a Christian conception of the person nor a naturalistic one, both of which have metaphysical assumptions. However, if it were, as perhaps Jonsen interpreted it, it could not be adopted in *a* common, sharable morality. In this context, 'person' is simply synonymous with agent and includes not only mature individuals, but also, in a dispositional sense, children and incapacitated ones (disabled persons) and vulnerable populations (preterm babies, prisoners etc.) with diminished autonomy. It is an open question whether non-human animals are capable of rule-following behaviour. Now, according to the Belmont Report, "An autonomous person is an individual capable of deliberation about personal goals and of acting under the direction of such deliberation. To respect autonomy is to give weight to autonomous persons' considered opinions and choices while refraining from obstructing their actions unless they are clearly detrimental to others." Note the interconnections between autonomy and non-maleficence, so an autonomous action cannot cause harm to others. Autonomy has then clear *limits* and it is not an absolute principle always overriding beneficence. I will re-examine this point when

---

[17] Downie, R. S. and Telfer, E., *Respect for Persons*, (New York: Schocken Books, 1970), 23.

discussing some *variations* of the Belmont Report, especially Beauchamp and Childress' principlism, but also subsequent important work in the normative foundations of bioethics as represented by Engelhardt's autonomism and Pellegrino's beneficence-in-trust model in the next chapter.

At this juncture, it becomes clear that we need a new meta-bioethical analysis of 'respect' in order to find out its proper object: either the person or simply autonomy. Many bioethicists hold that we need a robust moral notion such as respect for persons and not just for what an agent is capable of choosing and deciding (independently of further discussion about whether her choice is the right one). For them, a person is an entity with a special kind of value: dignity, which is not equivalent to price. This is a Kantian notion of the person. But a word may have the meaning that we choose to give to it. Thus, both the concept of 'person' and the notion of dignity may be naturalized. For instance, 'dignity' could refer to the social recognition of the worth of an individual (e.g., individuals with no job may, in this sense, have no dignity) or we may say that one wants to die with some dignity, meaning only: without suffering unnecessary pain. 'Dignity' means only a sense of one's own worth. In chapter 6, I will return to the principle of respect for persons.

I would now like to state another *prima facie* principle of the Belmont Report, namely:

b) Beneficence

Since there is no priority among the principles, beneficence is as important as respect for persons. On the principle of beneficence, the Belmont Report states:

> Persons are treated in an ethical manner not only by respecting their decisions and protecting them from harm, but also by making efforts to secure their wellbeing. Such treatment falls under the principle of beneficence. In this document, beneficence is understood in a stronger sense, as an obligation. Two general rules have been formulated as complementary expressions of beneficent actions in this sense: (1) do not harm and (2) maximize possible benefits and minimize possible harms.

This principle emphasizes the Hippocratic maxim which has been predominant in the history of Western medicine for more than two thousand years. Note, however, that the Hippocratic qualification, "above all" or "first" was left out in the "non-maleficence part" since all principles are considered valid *prima facie* only. This has huge implications, which will be discussed below. But, clearly, the principle states the obligation to provide a specific kind of care preventing harms and protecting the wellbeing of the subjects of scientific experimentation.

The Belmont Report had the clear intention of protecting vulnerable subjects of research/patients such as preterm babies. It established that effective ways of treating childhood diseases and fostering healthy development are benefits that serve to justify research involving children – even when individual research subjects are not direct beneficiaries. Going now back to our case, Baby 1 could have been regarded as a potential subject for further scientific research as a preterm (let us say, a teaching surgery to extract parts of her intestine, during which a new, experimental drug is used). Many bioethicists hold that the benefits of conducting research involving children are justified even when a particular individual is not the direct beneficiary. But supposing that the risks, for instance of an intestine transplantation, are more than minimal and there is no immediate prospect of it directly benefiting Baby 1 *herself*, should it be carried out to benefit the next generation? Should this operation be performed considering the possible benefits to children in the future (or, at least, the student doctor who would be able to perform better surgeries later in her professional life)? Isn't this a case of treating someone as a mere means, that is, as an object and not as a person?

This question reveals that we need a new meta-bioethical analysis of 'care' capable of showing us the proper object of caring and its appropriate relation to respect. I will provide such an analysis later, in chapter 4. Baby 1 is a hard case indeed and the Belmont Report contains, apparently, no way of resolving the conflict between the beneficence principle and the basic norm of respect for persons. That is why we need to look for a new balance between caring & respecting with the hope that philosophy can help to settle the issue and prevent cases such as Baby 1's from occurring again. The analyses of both care & respect may pave the way to redefining and reconceptualising them into a fundamental bioethical attitude: respectful care or caring respect.

Before arguing for that, let me now examine another principle of the Belmont Report:

c) Justice

The Belmont document deals also with the distribution of the burdens and benefits of scientific research, that is, with distributive justice. It states that the fundamental idea is fairness in distribution. This may be analysed in two main norms: *formally*, it requires that "equals ought to be treated equally," but then several questions arise: who counts as equal and who is different? What considerations justify a departure from equal distribution? For instance, should a hospital give priority to Baby 1 to the detriment of other patients who have already had a gratifying long life, but are terminally ill? How to use the limited resources in health care? Justice then requires also a *material* criterion for treating persons fairly. Thus, the Belmont Report enumerates five criteria:

i) to each person an equal share;
ii) to each person according to individual need;
iii) to each person according to individual effort;
iv) to each person according to societal contribution, and
v) to each person according to merit.

The referred to document does not state a procedure for deciding which criteria should be applied when they clash, although it seems to equate fairness with "what is deserved." Merit, however, is not the only material criterion that can be used, for instance, in selecting subjects for particular scientific research. Thus, the commissioners' "consensus" seems in fact worthless, since each of them could build up a theory of justice pushing for one material criterion to establish an unequal distribution ending up with a liberal or a communitarian or a libertarian political philosophy. As we will see in the next chapter, one way of overcoming this problem is to be crystal clear about which is the material criterion of justice most appropriate for the health care system.

No doubt principles of justice are the foundation of a fair health care system. Just to examine our case further, namely the Baby 1 story, consider that the health insurance plan (a form of M-care supplement) did not cover a transfer to other facilities where a transplant could, perhaps, have been done. If this was the case, it represents a clear disrespect for life and for the patient *herself*. Some bioethicists argue that society should pay the costs of such intensive care as required in this case. In the US, at that time, there were 48 million people without any health insurance. How can it be that the richest country in the world does not have enough money to save a life if it can be saved? If nothing else, the case of Baby 1 shows that it is necessary to support a universal health system like the one which exists in the UK and many other countries around the world including Brazil. It was only in 2010 that President Obama managed to push through a similar system, which could, however, be not enough to save babies in similar circumstances. Now, Baby 1's case also raises other questions of justice. For instance: is it fair, from a social point of view, to spend taxpayers' money on saving the life of a child who will, perhaps, have many disabilities, leaving thousands of poor children unassisted or dying? Common sense tells us that it is not, but scientific research shows that in fact we spend more on "normal" patients. This is why bioethics cannot be guided by common sense, but only by philosophical and scientific knowledge. I will discuss the best possible health system later, after analysing deeper the principles of justice.

Let me now make two ethico-philosophical points on the kind of normative bioethical approach that is provided by the Belmont Report. First, it seems clear that it tries to combine teleologically oriented principles, such as beneficence, with deontologically oriented ones, such as respect for persons and justice. This is interesting in overcoming traditional ways of doing ethics, but it also may be the cause of the tensions between caring and doing scientific research. As we saw in chapter 1, these tensions may turn into dilemmas and inaction. But if this is the best theoretical arrangement, then other approaches such as Engelhardt's view, namely that "most appeals to the principle of justice can be understood as being at root a concern with beneficence"[18] need to be reconsidered. Granted, principles of justice support the distribution of goods and there are right or wrong ways of doing it. The question is then which material criterion should be used? As we have seen, the Belmont Report does not give us a clear answer to this fundamental question. Thus, I will argue in this work that *basic needs* is the main material criterion that should be considered in issues surrounding distributive justice in the health care system.

Meta-ethically speaking, however, the Belmont Report is *intuitionist* in a Rawlsian sense, that is, it works with a plurality of norms denying that it is possible either to give more weight to one or to subsume them into a single principle. According to Rawls, intuitionism is:

> … the doctrine that there is an irreducible family of first principles which have to be weighed against one another by asking ourselves which balance, in our considered judgement, is the most just. Once we reach a certain level of generality, the intuitionist maintains that there exist no higher-order constructive criteria for determining the proper emphasis for the competing principles of justice.[19]

---

[18] Tristram Engelhardt, *The Foundations of Bioethics*, (Oxford: Oxford University Press, 1996), 121.

[19] John Rawls, *A Theory of Justice*, (Oxford: Oxford University Press, 1999), 30.

This intuitionist meta-ethics may, as we have seen in the first chapter, lead to dilemmas or arbitrary applications. We need to re-think this meta-ethical basis of special bioethics. This is a problem with the predominant principlist approach since it keeps the intuitionist framework and, consequently, is not capable of solving conflicts of principles. I will leave for the next chapter a more detailed discussion of the main changes the principlists made. That is to say, I will consider later what Beauchamp and Childress suggested, namely that a fundamental principle should be respect for *autonomy* and not respect for persons and their separation of the principle of *non-maleficence* from the principle of beneficence. Other characteristics of this view and its main variations will also be discussed in the next chapter.

I will now briefly examine some proposals for adding new principles to the Belmont's framework. It is worth starting by pointing out that even among those who worked closely with the National Commission and helped to formulate the Belmont Report there was no unanimity about the number and, more importantly, the contents of the fundamental principles. For instance, those working later in other commissions for the National Institutes of Health, argued that another basic norm was needed, namely "a fourth principle for contemporary research ethics, a *principle of respect for communities*."[20] According to this proposal, communities are not just aggregates of isolated individuals, but they have their own needs and interests. In the revision of the Belmont Report, this argument found support also from people working with different conceptual frameworks. To recognize this point, it is sufficient to recall here that feminists hold a "relational" account of agency and autonomy, which is basically communitarian, not individual autonomy.

Many other bioethicists have maintained that the principles derived from the Belmont Report are not sufficient to deal with complex bioethical problems. Some have argued for the *principle of solidarity*, which is considered a fundamental bioethical value in European countries. Solidarity for those in need would be a fundamental principle for many Brazilian bioethicists as well. A philosophical question is whether this principle would not be similar to that of beneficence. The principle of solidarity raises also questions related to paternalism. Moreover, during the Sixth World Congress of Bioethics in 2002, in Brasília, some argued that we need nowadays a "hard bioethics" capable of intervening in power relations to overcome many of the developing countries' problems, which

[20] Emmanuel, E. J. and Weijer, C. "Protecting Communities in Research: From a New Principle to Rational Protections." In: James Childress, *et al.* (eds), *Belmont Revisited*, (Washington: Georgetown University Press, 2005), 165f.

are mainly problems related to justice.[21] This is, however, a *political* problem regarding public policies based on the principles of justice. It is difficult to see how hard bioethics adds something substantive in normative terms while discussing justice. In this sense, a Rawlsian proposal incorporated by the principlists using the material criterion of basic needs seems more appropriate to deal with bioethical issues. I will return to this point in the next chapter while discussing models for a just health care system.

It has been suggested by some bioethicists referring to the Judeo-Christian tradition, that we need other principles as well, especially the already mentioned *principle of the sanctity of life*. In his book *Extreme Prematurity*, Geoffrey Miller describes this principle using these words:

> Human life is of infinite value. This in turn means that a piece of infinity is also infinite and a person who has a few moments of life is no less of value than a person who has sixty years to life … a handicapped individual is a perfect specimen when viewed as an ethical concept. The value is an absolute value. It is not relative to life expectancy, to state of health, or to usefulness to society.[22]

Recent attempts to work out a transcultural bioethical approach came to a similar conclusion adding respect for life among the basic bioethical norms. In one of the best anthologies on this subject, one can read: "Each contributor has been clear about the basic value of respect for life. And each has, in his own way, acknowledged the values of beneficence, autonomy, nonmaleficence, and justice."[23] Obviously, the question here is whether respect for life is a universal principle or just, by chance, a basic norm contingently accepted by most existing moral systems, that is, part of *the* common morality. The principle of the sanctity of life may, however, lead to a radical position in which taking life is always intrinsically wrong.

---

[21] Volnei Garrafa and Dora Porto "Bioética, Poder e Injustiça: Por uma Ética de Intervenção" in: Volnei, Garrafa and Leo, Pessini (eds.), *Bioética: Poder e Injustiça*, (São Paulo: Loyola/São Camilo, 2004), 25f. For a presentation of the main trends in Brazilian bioethics see: Leo Pessini and Christian de Paul de Barchifontaine "An X-Ray of Bioethics in Brazil: Pioneering Voices, Institutional and Educational Program and Perspectives". In: Leo Pessini *et al.* (eds.), *Ibero-American Bioethics: History and Perspectives*, (Dordrecht: Springer, 2010), 89-106.

[22] Geoffrey Miller, *Extreme Prematurity*, (New York: Cambridge University Press), 70.

[23] Edmund Pellegrino *et al.* (eds), *Transcultural Dimensions in Medical Ethics*, (Maryland: University Publishing Group, 1992), 11.

That is to say, the act of killing would never be morally correct. Thus, this principle might not agree, for instance, with allowing nonterminal, severely disabled infants, in our case a baby with no intestines, to die. This is counterintuitive. Moreover, there are circumstances where killing seems justified, for instance in self-defence, a just war, etc.

I will now propose, based on Dworkin's *Life's Dominion*, which argues that bioethical problems must be dealt with using the notion of the intrinsic value of life, the following principle*: revere life's inherent worth*. It fits well not only with special bioethics, but mainly with holistic bioethics. In order to understand this principle and its implications, we need first to analyse the concept of respect, distinguishing it from reverence, and this will be done in due course. It is necessary to point out here, however, that a Dworkinian principle, "revere life's inherent worth," differs from the sanctity of life principle in the sense that it is not absolute. That is to say, it allows for quality of life judgments. I will develop this principle in the last chapter.

Before making a critical assessment of these proposals, we need to discuss in a more detailed way the predominant normative theory, namely the approach based on the "four principles", also known, especially by its critics, as "principlism" and its variations, mainly autonomism and beneficence-in-trust. This is the task for the next chapter.

CHAPTER THREE

RETHINKING THE NORMATIVE BASIS OF SPECIAL BIOETHICS

In the previous chapter, I reconstructed the Belmont's normative framework based on the principles of respect for persons, beneficence and justice and its meta-ethical assumptions. In this chapter, I will first discuss the predominant normative theory in special bioethics, namely principlism, as expressed in the book *The Principles of Biomedical Ethics*. The main intention is to show that an intuitionist meta-ethical basis leads to conflicts in the application of basic norms and that this problem must be fixed. In the second section, I will examine two proposals for overcoming this difficulty by ranking one basic norm over the others, especially Engelhardt's defence of the priority of autonomy and Pellegrino's reformation of the Hippocratic tradition leading to the model of beneficence-in-trust. As we will see, these solutions are not satisfactory since the first leads to indifference or individualism and the second is in danger of running into some forms of paternalism. Thus, we need to look for better alternatives, which may be provided by re-analysing both care & respect leading to the concept of respectful care, which will be presented later.

3.1 The four principles approach

One of the first and most important departures from the Belmont Report, as we have seen, the "constitution" of special bioethics, which established the principles of respect for persons, beneficence and justice for scientific experimentation with human subjects, was made by Beauchamp and Childress. Having worked for the National Commission, Tom Beauchamp benefited from the discussions and results. As we have seen in the previous chapter, he actually wrote a draft of the document and contributed to the establishment of the principle of justice, but he left some material out of the final version. Then, together with James Childress, Beauchamp wrote the now highly acclaimed book *Principles of*

Biomedical Ethics, first printed in 1979, which has been published in seven different editions so far with major changes. Their approach is known as "principlism" or the "four principles approach". In this section, I will critically examine their views of the normative foundations of special bioethics.

Before engaging in the examination of "principlism," I would like to emphasize the strong influence it has nowadays. The four principles normative framework is the predominant approach both scientifically and academically around the world. It is also the ground for much legislation not only in the US where the Belmont Report still is a legal document. Principlism was, for instance, adopted in Brazil to give legitimacy to its bioethical and biosafety laws. Thus, Resolução 196/1996, now updated as 466/2012, regulating research involving human subjects, states that ethics in scientific investigations amounts to:

> a) freely given and informed consent of target-individuals and the protection of vulnerable groups and the legally disabled (*autonomy*). To that end, research involving human subjects must always preserve their dignity, respect their autonomy and defend them in their vulnerability;
>
> b) weighing risks and benefits, both actual and potential, individual and collective (*beneficence*), making a commitment to maximize benefits and minimize distress and risks;
>
> c) ensuring that predictable injury will be prevented (*non-maleficence*);
>
> d) social relevance of the research, with significant advantages to the research subjects and minimization of the burden to vulnerable individuals, which guarantees equal consideration of all interests involved and preserves the socio-humanitarian purpose of research (*justice and equality*).[1]

As can be seen, in Brazil, the official bioethical approach, despite the enormous influence of Catholic bioethicists such as Leo Pessini and Christian de Paul de Barchifontaine,[2] is principlism as developed by Beauchamp and Childress in *Principles of Biomedical Ethics*. Principlism was introduced into Brazilian legislation by Dr. William Saad Hossne, president of the CONEP - Comissão Nacional para a Ética na Pesquisa (National Commission for Ethics in Research), in 1996.

Let me start to analyse the four principles approach by comparing it with the Belmont Report itself. Now, without pretending to comment on

---

[1] A copy of the new document 466/2012 can be found here: http://conselho.saude.gov.br/resolucoes/2012/Reso466.pdf

[2] See Leo Pessini and Christian de Paul de Barchifontaine, *Problemas Atuais de Bioética*, (São Paulo: São Camilo/Edições Loyola, 2010).

all the changes to the several editions of the book *Principles of Biomedical Ethics*, let me here outline some that are important in recognizing the problems with the principlist approach itself. Some secondary variations are indicated in the footnotes. As we saw above regarding the Belmont Report, Beauchamp himself contributed to establishing one principle, namely that of *distributive* justice, while serving as a staff philosopher for the National Commission. Thus, instead of discussing at this point all the changes to the different editions in detail and their relations to various competing theories, it is worth pointing out the differences from the Belmont Report itself. According to some bioethicists, the Belmont Report and Beauchamp and Childress' book represent two different moral visions.

One of the major changes Beauchamp and Childress made in relation to the Belmont Report, maintained in all the different editions, was the introduction of the principle of respect for *autonomy* instead of respect for *persons*. They argued that "the concept of 'personhood' is so inherently contestable that we avoid it in this book insofar as possible. This is one reason, among others, that we shy away from the language of 'respect for persons' in this book."[3] Answering a critic on how *respect for persons* became *respect for autonomy*, the authors of *Principles of Biomedical Ethics* wrote:

> Obligations to respect autonomy do not extend to persons who cannot act in a sufficiently autonomous manner –and who cannot be rendered autonomous– because, for instance, they are immature, incapacitated, ignorant, coerced, or exploited. Infants, irrationally suicidal individuals, and drug-dependent patients are examples. This standpoint does not presume that these individuals are not owed moral respect. In our framework, they have a significant moral status … that obligates us to protect them from harm-causing conditions and to supply medical benefits.[4]

---

[3] Tom L. Beauchamp and James F. Childress, *Principles of Biomedical Ethics*, (New York/Oxford: Oxford University Press, 2013), 68.

[4] Tom L. Beauchamp and James F. Childress, *Principles of Biomedical Ethics*, (New York/Oxford: Oxford University Press, 2013), 108. Now, in the *first* edition of the book, published in 1979, just a year after the Belmont Report, the authors set out the following starting points: first, they used only two major traditional ethical approaches right at the beginning of their book, namely *utilitarianism* and *deontological theories*, with special mention of Mill and Kant, but also of Ross, Frankena and others, to arrive at their theory (pp.21-55); second, they presented a diagram for moral justification in this way "judgments and action → rules → principles → ethical theories" (p.5), and this was used to explain, justify and illustrate the application of the middle level principles assuming a *top-down* model

The explanation given by Beauchamp and Childress seems unconvincing. Contestability is not a sufficient reason to abandon the principle of respect for persons. Thus, after arguing that the language of "respect for persons" is too unclear regarding what is to be respected and how it is to be respected, Beauchamp and Childress focused instead on autonomous *choices* and autonomous *actions*. In their own words: "To respect an autonomous agent is to acknowledge their right to hold views, to make choices, and to take actions based on personal values and beliefs."[5] But this is not all that the principle of respect for autonomy requires since they recognize positive obligations and explicitly agree that "as Kantians have argued, the demand that we treat others as ends requires that we assist them in achieving their ends and foster their capacities as agents, not merely that we avoid treating them solely as means to our ends."[6] Thus, they seem to assume a Kantian notion of *autonomy* and, more importantly, of person, which is completely different from that of a Millian autonomous individual perhaps conceived naturalistically.[7] A Kantian notion of person involves the notion of dignity, that is, a concept most of the time characterized in metaphysical terms. There is no doubt that to respect a person's decision is to value her as an end in herself, but this point relates to the Humanity Formula of Kant's Categorical Imperative and not to the Autonomy Formula.[8] I doubt, therefore, that Beauchamp and Childress have sufficiently clarified their own views, and this tension seems due to

---

(deductivist); third, autonomy, beneficence, nonmaleficence and justice (chapters 3-6) were explicitly called "principles" departing from the Belmont Report not only in changing the principle from respect for persons to respect for autonomy, but also dismembering the principle of beneficence into two (non-maleficence and beneficence); fourth, there was a chapter on "Ideals, Virtues and Integrity" (chap. 8), but not an explicit engagement with *virtue ethics*.

[5] Tom L. Beauchamp and James F. Childress, *Principles of Biomedical Ethics*, (New York/Oxford: Oxford University Press, 2013), 106.

[6] Tom L. Beauchamp and James F. Childress, *Principles of Biomedical Ethics*, (New York/Oxford: Oxford University Press, 2013), 107.

[7] For a discrimination between a Millian 'individual autonomy' and a Kantian 'principled autonomy' see: Onora O'Neill, *Autonomy and Trust in Bioethics*, (Cambridge: Cambridge University Press, 2002), 73s.

[8] This formula of the Categorical Imperative asserts: "So act that you use humanity, whether in your own person or in the person of any other, always at the same time as an end, never merely as a means." Immanuel Kant, *Groundwork of the Metaphysics of Morals* (4: 429), in: Immanuel Kant, *Practical Philosophy*, (Cambridge: Cambridge University Press, 2008), 80. This formulation is the basis for an ethics based on universal respect as developed by Tugendhat, Dworkin, Darwall etc. I will return to this point in the next chapter.

the utilitarianism accepted by the first philosopher and the Rossian deontology subscribed to by the co-author. By insisting on self-determination, they seem to endorse a Millian notion of individual autonomy only as it becomes clear at the end of the section "The Triumph or Failure of Respect for Autonomy?": "health professionals should almost always inquire about their patients' wishes to receive information and to make decisions, and they should not assume that because a patient belongs to a particular community or culture, he or she affirms that community's worldview and values."[9] This is certainly a preferentialist approach to wellbeing. Should this be applied in the case of Baby 1? The results would be predictable since health professionals would give patients what they wish and this is not what a Kantian notion of autonomy would require at all.

To clarify this point, let me reconstruct Beauchamp and Childress' "Three-condition Theory of Autonomy." As I have already pointed out, they focused on autonomous *choices* or on particular autonomous *acts* rather than the general capacity for deliberating since even full competent persons may fail to take autonomous decisions, for instance, when a person signs an informed consent form without reading it. Now, according to Beauchamp and Childress, a particular action is autonomous if it satisfies the following three conditions: i) intentionality; ii) understanding; and iii) noncontrol.[10] This is an attempt to present a *conceptual analysis* of autonomous *action,* spelling out the necessary and sufficient conditions for applying a concept. A significant merit of their work is, certainly, to try to practice this kind of method bringing more clarity to the issues they discuss, which is also exemplified in their analysis of the obligation a health professional has to rescue a patient in danger of losing her life.[11] I will not comment on their explanations of these three conditions of autonomous action, which seem clear enough, but I will argue that they are not *sufficient* to impute an action to an agent. Thus, I think that even after all the editions and corrections, Beauchamp and Childress did not present us with a clear analysis of autonomous *action*. That is to say, an agent A

[9] Tom L. Beauchamp and James F. Childress, *Principles of Biomedical Ethics*, (New York/Oxford: Oxford University Press, 2013), 110.

[10] Tom L. Beauchamp and James F. Childress, *Principles of Biomedical Ethics*, (New York/Oxford: Oxford University Press, 2013), 104.

[11] Differently from their analysis of autonomous action, Beauchamp and Childress seem to present a successful analysis of the necessary and *sufficient* conditions to say that a person X has a *prima facie* obligation of beneficence towards Y. See: Tom Beauchamp and James Childress, *Principles of Biomedical Ethics*, (New York/Oxford: Oxford University Press, 2013), 206-7.

may have the intention and the understanding needed to perform p (e.g., signing an informed consent form), and be negatively free to do so, but p may never be the case. That is to say, even if all the conditions were satisfied, they would not conjointly be sufficient to make p true. Beauchamp and Childress seem to have no reason, therefore, to complain about the use of the principle of respect for persons since their theory of autonomous action offers no better alternative.

Having pointed out that Beauchamp and Childress focus on autonomous action and not on autonomy generally (e.g., as self-imposition of laws) and having criticised their analysis, I would like to reconstruct how they formulate the principle itself. The norm of respect for autonomy can be stated in a *positive* sense requiring both respectful treatment in disclosing information and actions that foster autonomous decision-making, and in a *negative* way prescribing that one must respect individuals' views and rights so long as their thoughts and actions do not seriously harm other persons.[12] From this universal norm, a set of particular rules was drawn up in order *to specify* its contents: i) tell the truth; ii) respect the privacy of others; iii) protect confidential information; iv) obtain consent for interventions with patients; v) when asked, help others make important decisions. This is an application of the *method of specification* referred to above. Some of these rules can be extracted from the principle, but it is doubtful whether all of them can be deduced from it. For instance, how can we show that telling the truth is something that follows from respect for autonomous action? Again, it seems that Beauchamp and Childress have a more robust notion of autonomy not clearly enunciated.

There are other problems as well. For instance, if autonomy is merely a capacity subject to degrees (e.g., noncontrol), then the problem is how to establish that a person is acting in a fully autonomous way. It seems that it remains within the doctor's power to say whether an individual is autonomous or not. Thus, since respect is, as we will see later, related to a person's rights and autonomous decision-making is just one right among others, it is perhaps necessary to keep the principle *respect for persons* in order to avoid the dark side of the doctor's power. We may realize the limits of autonomy if, for instance, a father argues that he has "the right" to refuse conventional medical treatment and the right to choose alternative cures (for example, based on herbs, with no scientific evidence of being beneficial) for his son's lymphatic cancer, but that "right" may be

---

[12] Tom L. Beauchamp and James F. Childress, *Principles of Biomedical Ethics*, (New York/Oxford: Oxford University Press, 2013), 107.

overlooked to prevent harm to the child himself. Thus, it seems clear that, in the case of Baby 1, the health team is under no obligation to give to parents everything they want. The preferentialist view seems simply wrong or has clear limits. This is an error most autonomists make, namely they do not realize that the principle of autonomy is *limited* by the principle of non-maleficence. I will argue for this point in the next section.

To avoid misunderstandings, it is necessary to point out that the principle of respect for autonomy is not, according to principlism, *prior* to the others.[13] That is to say, the authors of the *Principles of Biomedical Ethics* retain the intuitionist meta-ethics of the Belmont Report denying that the principle of autonomy is more fundamental. In fact, it was only Tristram Engelhardt, in *The Foundations of Bioethics*, who gave absolute priority to individual autonomy over all other principles. That is why his view is known as "autonomism". Finally, it is worth stressing that Beauchamp and Childress do not appeal to a meta-principle to guide the application of the middle level principles such as the Categorical Imperative or the Utilitarian Principle. This may be one of the sources of their difficulties in avoiding dilemmas in the application of the middle level principles of respect for autonomy, non-maleficence, beneficence and justice.

Having noted an ambiguity in the principle of respect for autonomy and having compared it with the principle of respect for persons, I would like to make the following remark: if the principle of respect for persons as stated in the Belmont Report uses a Christian notion of personhood (as some commissioners argued), then it cannot be used as a universal principle, and Beauchamp and Childress may be right in trying to move to individual autonomy given that we must assume an agnostic attitude regarding metaphysical issues. But this can also be done using the concept of 'person' in a non-metaphysical way. For example, we may define a

---

[13] Tom L. Beauchamp and James F. Childress, *Principles of Biomedical Ethics*, (New York/Oxford: Oxford University Press, 2013), p. ix. This is true of all editions, including the *second*, which does not exhibit any significant changes in relation to the first. Now, in the *third* edition, the main changes are the following: i) introduction of large bodies of entirely new material throughout every chapter, including various topics such as AIDS and artificial nutrition and hydration (also substantial discussion of each principle, for instance, justice from a libertarian, an egalitarian etc. point of view and the introduction of the right to a decent minimum of health care); ii) the bioethical cases are discussed in the text itself and no longer at the end; iii) the authors dropped the appendix of codes (Hippocratic Oath, Declaration of Geneva, AMA's Principles of Medical Ethics, A Patient's Bill of Rights, The Nuremberg Code, Declaration of Helsinki, Code for Nurses), which had appeared in the two previous editions.

person as a rule-following being, a bearer of rights and obligations only. I will return to this definition later.

A second significant change regarding the principles of the Belmont Report promoted by Beauchamp and Childress was to detach the principle of non-maleficence from beneficence. Even common sense morality seems to tell us that when there is nothing good we can do, we must do nothing. Non-maleficence is a fundamental principle of the law also, especially penal law. According to Beauchamp and Childress, the Hippocratic tradition in medicine had already made it clear that a health professional must "*primum* (first)" do no harm. As we will see, this does not give logical priority to non-maleficence, that is, it doesn't mean that non-maleficence has absolute priority or that one must not "at least" do more good than a little harm. It is always worth remembering that this remains a *prima facie* principle in their view. This basic norm "you ought not to inflict evil or harm" justifies several particular obligations: i) do not kill; ii) do not cause pain or suffering; iii) do not incapacitate; iv) do not cause offence; v) do not deprive others of the goods of life. We have here a web of norms relating to a principle which has a justificatory role leading to particular rules to guide action. This web of norms, composed of principles and rules, must *cohere*. However, if the concept of 'harm' is not clarified, many questions remain. To recall our case, the Baby 1 story, one may wonder what exactly *do no harm* amounts to: withholding or withdrawing treatment? Directly taking the patient's life or letting her die?

Before trying to answer these questions and given that there seems to be a continuum between non-maleficence and beneficence and that both can apparently be reduced to care, let me now analyse another basic norm. The principle of beneficence, which simply refers to the obligation to act for the benefit of others as the Belmont Report itself stipulates, supports, according to Beauchamp and Childress, another set of moral rules closely related to the principle of non-maleficence. They are: i) protect and defend the rights of others; ii) prevent harm from occurring to others; iii) remove conditions that will cause harm to others; iv) help persons with disabilities; v) rescue persons in danger. It seems that these two principles, beneficence and non-maleficence, can be unified under a single principle or notion, but there is a clear difference between intentionally refraining from actions that cause harm, a clear obligation in health care and, for instance, trying to prevent harm or removing it from happening. In any case, *caring* for someone requires both doing no harm and acting for the person's benefit.

To say that we must act for the benefit of others is a simple basic norm, but the open question is: what is the good to be done and, perhaps more importantly, who says what counts as good or not? If we now relate the principle of beneficence with the principle of respect for autonomy, then it seems clear that Beauchamp and Childress would say that it is the patient or the subject of scientific research who has the final word. That is to say, according to Beauchamp and Childress, "to respect autonomous agents is to acknowledge their right to hold views, to make choices, and to take actions based on their *values and beliefs*," (italics added).[14] Therefore, it seems that it is the patient's own conception of the good that must be respected. This is a preferentialist theory of the good, standing in opposition to other models such as Pellegrino's beneficence-in-trust and the rational theory of welfare as proposed by Stephen Darwall based on an Aristotelian thesis. I will analyse Pellegrino's model in the next section and Darwall's theory in the next chapter. But at this juncture it is necessary to point out that if we relate the good to some worldview, then it seems clear, assuming that agnosticism is the most reasonable stance regarding metaphysical issues, that Beauchamp and Childress are right in holding that it is up to autonomous agents to choose freely according to their values and beliefs what they want to do and how they want to live. A person is free to choose to keep the worldview she was educated to have or to change to a different one she finds more suitable for her. It may be possible, however, to find particular good things (just for example's sake, health), which are constitutive of *any* worldview. Thus, assuming agnosticism does lead to pluralism about worldviews, but not necessarily to ethical relativism in all domains of life, we need then *a* common, sharable morality capable of establishing a moral minimum for any person belonging to any worldview. I will develop this argument in the next chapter, but before doing that let me say something regarding justice as defended by the principlists.

In relation to the supposed principles of justice, Beauchamp and Childress apparently made no significant progress compared to the Belmont Report.[15] First, they only reiterated that there is a *formal* principle

[14] Tom L. Beauchamp and James F. Childress, *Principles of Biomedical Ethics*, (New York/Oxford: Oxford University Press, 2013), 106.

[15] In the *fourth* edition of Beauchamp and Childress' book, the changes are the following: in chapter 1, the authors added entirely new sections on method, justification and truth, specifying and balancing principles, and they discuss the place of principles in *the* common morality; in chapter 2, they developed new sections on liberal individualism, communitarianism, the ethics of care, casuistry, and principle-based, common-morality theories; in chapter 6, in the fair opportunity section, the authors added a subsection concerning distributing health care on the basis of gender and race. Moreover, other major sections were added on the justification of assistance in dying, the value and quality of life and

traditionally attributed to Aristotle, which states that equals must be treated equally (and unequals must be treated differently). This is a minimal requirement that can be accepted by almost all theories of justice. Second, they repeat the list of candidates to formulate *material* principles, for example need, merit, etc., which had already appeared in the Belmont document itself. In their last edition of the book *Principles of Biomedical Ethics*, Beauchamp and Childress, based on four traditional theories of justice (utilitarian, libertarian, communitarian and egalitarian) and two recent ones (capabilities and wellbeing), state six *material* principles of justice respectively:

i) to each person according to rules and actions that maximize social utility;
ii) to each person a maximum of liberty and property resulting from the exercise of liberty rights and participation in fair free-market exchanges;
iii) to each person according to principles of fair distribution derived from conception of the good developed in moral communities;
iv) to each person an equal measure of liberty and equal access to the goods in life that every rational person values;
v) to each person the means necessary for the exercise of capabilities essential for a flourishing life;
vi) to each person the means necessary for the realization of core dimension of wellbeing.[16]

As can be seen, they apparently do not improve in relation to the Belmont Report, except by adding new material criteria for distribution. In fact,

---

rationing through priorities in the health care budget. In chapter 8, a new section on virtues in professional roles explicitly mentions four virtues, namely compassion, discernment, trustworthiness and integrity.

[16] Tom L. Beauchamp and James F. Childress, *Principles of Biomedical Ethics*, (New York/Oxford: Oxford University Press, 2013), 253. The *fifth* edition does not exhibit any significant changes considering the previous one. In the *sixth* edition, published in 2009, the main changes are the following: i) chapter 3, on the subject of moral status, is entirely new; ii) expansions of the common morality in chapters 1 and 10 (common morality as universal morality); iii) in chapter 7, on justice, the authors introduced a new discussion on globalization and philosophical thinking about the global order; iv) in Chapter 2, ethics of care was revised as a form of virtue ethics (the virtue of caring); v) the authors paid closer attention to the precautionary principle; vi) practical reasoning is no longer thought of in terms of top-down or bottom-up only, but "reflective equilibrium" is defended as an integrating model.

Beauchamp and Childress manifest a "sceptical caution" arguing that "no single moral principle is capable of addressing all problems of justice" and that very likely "there has never been a political state or a world order fashioned *entirely* on one and only one of the several theories of justice."[17] Their way out was to embrace aspects of *all* theories of justice at once.

To be fair, however, Beauchamp and Childress did more recently make an effort to contribute to the understanding of at least one particular theory, that is, the *egalitarian* theory of distributive justice, especially related to issues of health care and public health resources. Based on a Rawlsian fair opportunity principle, they argued for the right to a *decent minimum* of health care for all. To better scrutinize this proposal, it is necessary to briefly reconstruct Rawls' principles of justice.

In his now classic book *A Theory of Justice*, first published in 1971, John Rawls argues that in the original position (a thought experiment designed to guarantee an impartial point of view), under a veil of ignorance (persons do not know their place in society, their personal features etc., but do know the circumstances of justice, economic laws etc.), the parts would *contract* two principles of justice in this *lexical* order:

> (i) each person is to have an equal right to the most extensive total system of equal basic liberties compatible with a similar system of liberty for all;
> (ii) social and economic inequalities are to be arranged so that they are both: (a) to the greatest benefit of the least advantaged, consistent with the just savings principle, and (b) attached to offices and positions open to all under conditions of fair equality of opportunity.[18]

This is the core of the theory of justice as *fairness*.

Despite the fact that Rawls himself did not apply these principles to health care institutions, some philosophers have explored his ideas placing health as a primary good. In this direction, Norman Daniels[19] made an important contribution arguing that health is a condition for fair equality of

---

[17] Tom L. Beauchamp and James F. Childress, *Principles of Biomedical Ethics*, (New York/Oxford: Oxford University Press, 2013), 262. Since I have mainly used this *seventh* edition in this work, I will not indicate more secondary changes in the footnotes.

[18] John Rawls, *A Theory of Justice*, (Oxford: Oxford University Press, 1999), 266. For critical studies of Rawls' theory of justice as fairness see: Norman Daniels, *Reading Rawls*, (Stanford: Stanford University Press, 1989).

[19] See Norman Daniels, *Just Health Care*, (Cambridge: Cambridge University Press, 1995).

opportunity, which was later assimilated by Beauchamp and Childress. I believe, however, that the principle of fair equality of opportunity is better applied in other areas, for instance, in education. Thus, I will from now on argue that a more promising alternative would be to consider health care in terms of the *basic needs principle*. In his later work *Political Liberalism*, first published in 1993, John Rawls accepts that “the first principle covering the equal basic rights and liberties may easily be preceded by a lexically prior principle requiring that citizen’s *basic needs* be met, at least insofar as their being met is necessary for citizens to understand and to be able fruitfully to exercise those rights and liberties,” (italics added).[20] Consequently, a more promising Rawlsian health care system would be based on satisfying basic needs as a material criterion for distributive justice.

The right to a decent minimum generates, according to Beauchamp and Childress, a *mixed* health care system composed of two main tiers: “enforced social coverage for basic and catastrophic health needs (tier 1), together with voluntary private coverage for other health needs and desires (tier 2).”[21] This mixed health system is described in this way:

(i) *first tier* (universal access to basic services): cover at least public health protections and preventive care, primary care, acute care, and special social services for those with disabilities;
(ii) *second tier*: luxury hospital rooms and optional, cosmetic dental work are available for purchase at personal expense though private health insurance or direct payment.

The authors recognize that the model is purely programmatic until society delineates the decent minimum in operational terms. They hope, however, that it may lead to a “compromise among various theories of justice”.[22] I am skeptical whether libertarianists would subscribe to it, but the mixed health system is a good *model* for rethinking both the American system

---

[20] John Rawls, *Political liberalism*, (New York: Columbia University Press, 1993), 7. For a guide to the communitarian/liberal debate, including a study of Rawls' main changes from *A Theory of Justice* to *Political Liberalism*, see: Stephen Mulhall and Adam Swift, *Liberals & Communitarians*, (Oxford: Wiley-Blackwell, 1996). See also: Shlomo Avineri and Avner de-Shalit (eds.), *Communitarianism and Individualism*, (Oxford: Oxford University Press, 1995).

[21] Tom L. Beauchamp and James F. Childress, *Principles of Biomedical Ethics*, (New York/Oxford: Oxford University Press, 2013), 273.

[22] Tom L. Beauchamp and James F. Childress, *Principles of Biomedical Ethics*, (New York/Oxford: Oxford University Press, 2013), 273.

based on private health insurance and the British/Brazilian universal systems, which cannot provide everything for everyone. Of course, the distinction between what are *basic* needs or not is also controversial, but the decent minimum must at least satisfy them and the list of things covered in the first tier seems a good starting point. Since this is an important issue anyway, I will return to it when discussing further questions of justice in the health care system. I will below introduce a new bioethical case to illustrate how complex these issues are.

Having presented the main substantial normative changes Beauchamp and Childress introduced into the Belmont bioethical framework and having pointed out that they kept the intuitionist meta-ethics of the Belmont Report, let me now discuss two other approaches that were somehow influenced by that document, but that looked for a different way of avoiding the meta-ethical difficulties of principlism. These are the views of Engelhardt's autonomism and Pellegrino's beneficence-in-trust model, which rank one principle above the others. As we will see, both still present problems. We need, consequently, to continue looking for better solutions.

3.2 Autonomism *versus* Beneficence-in-Trust

Before discussing these two bioethical theories, which left behind the intuitionist meta-ethics of the Belmont Report accepted by the principlists Beauchamp and Childress, let me introduce another bioethical case. It will help us to critically analyse whether autonomism or beneficence-in-trust are better alternatives to the four principles approach.

Consider then another real life bioethical case:

> Baby 2 was born in the HU at the U. of B., Brazil, on 02/06/2007, weighing 535gr. She was 29cm long. The gestational age would be 22 weeks considering GPA –gestational postmenstrual age– and 24 weeks using the Ballard method. Two days previously, her mother had PRM (premature rupture of membranes) and two options were given to the family: i) to induce birth (which could mean abortion); ii) to wait some more days so that the foetus could be saved. Despite the fact that they chose the second course of action, the mother had an infection (very common in those circumstances) and the medical team induced birth to protect the mother's life. Baby 2 was born alive, but left to die. After much crying, she was taken to the NICU under mechanical ventilation and PN (parenteral nutrition). She had several problems: anaemia; renal failure; hypothermia; multiple organ dysfunction; heavy bleeding; she was also pneumothorax and so on. Baby 2 responded well to all treatments. On 17/07/2007, she was transferred to the NICU of Hospital Y for a surgical

> intervention to close an arterial channel. The procedure was successful and Baby 2 went back to the hospital of the U. of B. on 22/07/2007. She left the facility on 26/10/2007 and the costs were covered by SUS (Sistema Único de Saúde), the Brazilian universal coverage health system. At two years of age, Baby 2 needs a cochlear transplant and has immunity problems.

This case can be regarded as a story intended to save the mother's life (interrupting the gestation was not the real declared intention), which turned into a happy story. However, it is worth remembering that a baby is considered premature until she reaches 2 years old and may even develop several complications as a teenager or later in her life.

Some of the bioethical questions of this case are: was abortion an intended effect or a merely foreseen one? This is a distinction that Catholic moralists take seriously and we must remember that Catholicism is still Brazil's predominant religion despite being a secular state and a pluralist society, but is it philosophically relevant and sustainable? On the one hand, in Brazil, there are two circumstances when abortion is permitted by law: to save the mother's life, the official reason invoked in the case narrated above, and if the pregnancy resulted from rape. On the other hand, in the US, after the famous case *Roe versus Wade*, a mother may abort her pregnancy for any reason up to the "point at which the foetus becomes 'viable.'" The Court defined *viable* as being potentially able to live outside the mother's womb, albeit with artificial aid. Viability is usually placed at about seven months (28 weeks) but may occur earlier, even at 24 weeks. Baby 1 was at the edge of viability. Now, in the case of Baby 2, in normal circumstances, she would never be legally subject to an abortion in Brazil. Do these cultural differences between Brazil's predominantly Catholic morality (supposedly, more conservative) and the US's majority Protestant morality (supposedly, more liberal) really matter in resolving either of the two cases? Does *cultural relativism*, that is, the fact that there is a plurality of moral systems prove *meta-ethical relativism*, namely the idea that two opposite moral judgments may be both right (abortion in the first trimester is wrong in Brazil, but okay in the US)? I will return to some of these ethical questions in the next chapter on the idea of a common morality and in chapter 5.

Other questions surrounding this case can be put in the following way: shouldn't the health team apply the *principle of non-maleficence*, which may have some kind of priority over *beneficence* given the very high probability of Baby 2 becoming a severely disabled person and not try to save her? What kind of method was applied to balance the risks and benefits of proceeding with the surgery to save the baby? Are methods such as cost-effectiveness analysis (CEA) or cost-benefit analysis (CBA) applicable here? Can a human life have a price or are persons entities with *dignity* and not quantitative value? What about the risk-benefit analysis (RBA), how can we determine what constitutes a risk and its probability in this case: minimal, reasonable, high risk? Was the surgery in the Baby 2 case an ordinary or an extraordinary treatment? Was it an optional treatment or an obligatory one? Wouldn't aggressive obstetric management or intensive care produce more harms than benefits for Baby 2? Wouldn't it be better to allow Baby 2 simply to die?

These questions give rise to more ethical issues: what kind of *quality-of-life* will Baby 2 have? Preterm babies normally turn out to be children with severe illnesses or serious disabilities. Society and in particular families pay a high cost to keep them alive and functioning. Is it just in extreme cases such as Tay-Sachs or Lesch-Nyham diseases that it may be permissible to kill or to let the babies die, or also with some forms of Down syndrome? In Brazil, there is now a jurisprudence allowing abortion in the case of an anencephalic baby, but why not in other similar cases, microcephaly for instance? How can we determine what it means to be able to participate in "significant human experiences," a concept sometimes used to justify saving ELBW babies? Baby 2 was a seriously ill newborn, so is it justified to say that because her quality of life would be low and that the intervention would produce more harm than benefit, caregivers are justified in withholding treatment? Is the concept "quality of life" a purely descriptive one, based on facts and medical requirements, or is it also a normative one? Is QALYs (Quality-Adjusted Life-Years), as it is used in universal systems such as the NHS in the UK, a reliable method of evaluation and sufficient to determine whether a person should live or die?

Before trying to answer some of these questions (many more certainly can be raised), let me point out that the Hospital at the U. of B., in Brazil, is also a teaching and research facility that belongs to the network of public hospitals administrated by federal universities. This public system seems to be based on *solidarity,* a principle many Brazilians, perhaps following European values more than American ones, think should be added to the basic norms in bioethics. This means that all the costs were paid by the taxpayer (around three hundred thousand reais). Is this fair from a social point of view in a country where so many children still die due to a lack of proper nutrition and sanitation and, for instance, where the Zika virus is producing a generation of abnormal babies?

By comparing these two cases or stories, what can we learn from a bioethical point of view? There are, of course, philosophical questions, for instance, whether by starting from different cultural backgrounds we need to reaffirm existing pluralism and even some sort of (descriptive) relativism: perhaps the two cases have nothing in common and the different outcomes prove that no universal principle applies to both as casuists argue. After all, each case is different. Or, on the contrary, should these two cases, as any other case indeed, be judged by the same moral principles? For instance, it may be perhaps necessary to assume a first bioethical principle, which can be referred to as the non-maleficence one: *primum*, that is, above all and before anything else, do not cause more harms than benefits. But a relevant question related to non-maleficence is this: is *harm* susceptible to cultural variations? Can we cause harm to a Navajo, for instance, by disclosing information about a disease? Can the Hippocratic principle be justified *a priori* or is it just a transcultural one? Can a different principle such as respect for *autonomy* trump all other principles including non-maleficence?

What about the arbitrary application of these principles, for instance, if it is true that US society is more individualist, wouldn't a doctor put more stress on the *prima facie* principle of individual autonomy while in Brazil, supposedly a country with more emphasis on solidarity, a doctor would instead put more weight on the *prima facie* principle of beneficence? Can we avoid such arbitrary applications and their relativistic implications by finding a kind of metanorm, an axiom such as the Categorical Imperative or the Utility Principle or any other? I will answer these questions in chapter 5, after discussing autonomism and the beneficence-in-trust model.

I will start by analysing the view called "autonomism," which is in some respects another variation of the Belmont Report because it deals with the same fundamental norms. The already mentioned bioethicst Tristram Engelhardt is the best known proponent of the autonomist approach, that is, of the view that autonomy is the *first principle* of bioethics. Now, US bioethics is normally seen as being based on individualistic assumptions, which are in the background of a strong defence of the primacy of the principle of autonomy, the so called "all-American value". As Shannon says, "autonomy celebrates the hardy individualism for which our country is famous."[23] According to some bioethicists, autonomy is the cornerstone of US bioethics. As we have seen in the previous chapter, Engelhardt was the proponent of two "crisp" principles accepted by the commissioners, the first being respect for free

[23] Thomas A. Shannon, *An Introduction to Bioethics*, (New York: Paulist Press, 1997), 25. For a further discussion on the "The American Ethics" see: Albert Jonsen, *The Birth of Bioethics*, (New York/Oxford, Oxford University Press, 1998), 389

moral agents. Thus, he is the most forceful defender of autonomy in its individualistic assumptions. As we will see, Engelhardt clearly is a bioethicist who thinks that care is, in some sense, agent-relative, that is, one must do to others *their* good; what they think is good for them.

I will now examine carefully this preferentialist view, relating it to the cases we have been examining. In his book *The Foundations of Bioethics*, first published in 1986, Engelhardt argued that the basic principles of bioethics should be understood as resolving moral disputes in secular, *pluralistic* societies where no unique moral sense can be established. He is arguably the philosopher who most explored the implications of pluralism, particularly for bioethics. According to him, "laws protecting human research subjects against being used in experimentation without their consent carry moral authority in that they are grounded in the very notion of protecting the peaceable community. They spring from the notion of the morality of mutual respect."[24] Respect then is, according to Engelhardt, *sufficient* to ground morality. To make sense of this morality of mutual respect, in the first edition of *The Foundations of Bioethics*, he holds the following version of the *principle of autonomy*:

> Authority for actions involving others in a secular pluralistic society is derived from the free consent of those involved. As a consequence,
>
> i) Without such consent there is no authority;
> ii) Actions against such authority are blameworthy in the sense of placing a violator outside the moral community in general, and making licit (but not obligatory) retaliatory, defensive, or punitive force by members of any particular moral community.[25]

This is supposedly the *cardinal* principle of bioethics, which justifies implicit and explicit consent for research involving human subjects in scientific experimentation. The maxim of this principle is "do not do to others that which they would not have done unto them, and do for them that which one has contracted to do." The principle of autonomy grounds what is called "morality as mutual respect" only.

Now, the principle of beneficence, according to Engelhardt, asserts that the goal of moral action is the achievement of goods and the avoidance of

---

[24] Tristram Engelhardt, *The Foundations of Bioethics*, (New York/Oxford: Oxford University Press, 1996), 122. Engelhardt's general explanations of the principles of bioethics can be found in chapter 3 of his just referred to book. For a comprehensive study of Engelhardt's views see: Kevin Wm Wildes, *Moral Acquaintances*, (Notre Dame: Notre Dame University, 2000).

[25] Tristram Engelhardt, *The Foundations of Bioethics*, (New York/Oxford: Oxford University Press, 1986), 119.

harms within a particular moral community, for instance, a Christian one. Engelhardt discusses abortion, assisted reproduction, cloning, withholding or withdrawing treatment, assisted suicide and euthanasia from the perspective of moral friends in *The Foundations of Christian Bioethics*. But in a secular pluralist society, no unique ordering of goods and harms can be achieved. Therefore, there is no general content-full principle of beneficence for a public morality. Moral strangers need to contract particular forms of cooperation, for instance, in participating or not in scientific experimentation as subjects of particular tests. Actions against beneficence, however, are blameworthy in the sense of placing the violator outside the context of any particular moral community. More importantly, the principle of beneficence leads to the following *maxim*: "Do to others their good." As can clearly be seen here, care is taken to provide agent-relative reasons for action since it is what the person *actually* says that is her good (what she desires, prefers, has interest in etc.) which establishes what is good for her. This is clearly a preferentialistic view. I will discuss whether reasons based on care are agent-relative or agent-neutral in the next chapter.

In the second edition of his book *The Foundations of Bioethics*, Engelhardt substitutes "free consent of those involved" for "permission." Now, the first bioethical principle is called "The principle of permission". Why this change? Perhaps there is no substantial difference except in semantics since the justification of the principle of permission remains the same:

> The principle of permission expresses the circumstance that authority for resolving moral disputes in a secular, pluralist society can be derived only from the agreement of the participants, since it cannot be derived from rational argument or common belief. Therefore, permission or consent is the origin of authority, and respect of the right of participants to consent is *the necessary condition* for the possibility of a moral community. The principle of permission provides the minimum grammar for secular moral discourse. It is an inescapable as the interest of persons in blaming and praising with justification and resolving issues with moral authority (italics added).[26]

The first principle of Engelhardt's bioethics can be derived only from the agreement of the participants in the moral disputes. Thus, consent is the origin of authority. Moreover, respect for the right to consent is the

---

[26] Tristram Engelhardt, *The Foundations of Bioethics*, (New York/Oxford: Oxford University Press, 1996), 123.

necessary condition for the possibility of a moral community, but is it a *sufficient* one? How about a right to be cared for?[27]

It seems clear that such an account may lead to individualism if we take personal consent as the ultimate ground for morality. Engelhardt wants to avoid the association of autonomy with Kant because, in fact, his principle of permission is entirely Millian, that is, based on the idea of *individual self-determination*. John Stuart Mill wrote: "Over himself, over his own body and mind, the individual is sovereign."[28] This is certainly not autonomy in the Kantian sense of self-imposition of universal moral laws.

It is reasonable to say that Engelhardt overemphasizes the place of individual permission among the basic bioethical principles despite the fact that it seems to be a remedy for the intuitionist meta-ethical basis of the Belmont Report and classical principlism and their potentially arbitrary applications. He explicitly claims, as we will see soon, priority to the principle of consent. Now, if one gives absolute priority to respect for a particular person's actual preferences, choices etc., it may be empty of caring relationships, that is, it may lead to indifference and individualism. There is also the problem that what a particular individual prefers might not be *necessarily* what is always best for her from a caring point of view.

To recognize this point, compare Engelhardt's defence of the principle of permission with his justification of the principle of beneficence:

> the principle of beneficence reflects the circumstance that moral concerns encompass the pursuit of goods and the avoidance of harms. Since such disputes can be resolved in secular pluralistic societies only by an appeal to the principle of permission, the principle of permission is *conceptually prior* to the principle of beneficence. One can know when one is violating the morality of mutual respect, even when one cannot know, because of its lack of content, whether one is violating the principle of beneficence. However, recognition of the principle of beneficence provides the minimal characterizations of the content required for moral concerns (italics added).[29]

---

[27] I addressed this question personally to Engelhardt once in a congress in Florianópolis, and he emphatically denied that there is a right to be cared for. Afterwards, I wrote a comment on his defence of a morality of mutual respect arguing that to be cared for is a *necessary* condition to become an autonomous being (See: Dall'Agnol, 2012b).

[28] John S. Mill, *On Liberty and Other Writings*, (Cambridge: Cambridge University Press, 1994), 13.

[29] Tristram Engelhardt, *The Foundations of Bioethics*, (New York/Oxford: Oxford University Press, 1996), 123-4.

According to the author of *The Foundations of Bioethics*, even among "moral friends," that is, among those who *share* a particular moral system based on a specific worldview, some moral disagreement may exist. Obviously, among moral strangers, that is, those who do not share a particular moral system, disagreement is more common. Thus, in a peaceful, secular, pluralistic society, the principle of beneficence cannot carry much weight; otherwise, it leads to paternalism. Engelhardt believes that the principle of beneficence is not inescapable; it is not required for the moral life or even for a public bioethics.

Perhaps one may agree with this point, but it is difficult to accept that the *principle of justice* is, as Engelhardt holds, based on some concern with beneficence itself. He wrote: "Most appeals to the principle of justice can be understood as being at root a concern with beneficence."[30] That is to say, most views of justice are based on appeals to ideal distributions of goods presupposing particular views of the good life. The debates in bioethics are generally more concerned with *distributive* justice and Engelhardt seems no exception. On this particular issue, his view is that one may relate the distribution of goods to particular conceptions about what counts as beneficent. Thus, according to Engelhardt, "principles of justice that support the distribution of goods under a particular moral vision are special instances of attempting to do the good."[31] That is why justice is, in his opinion, an application of the principle of beneficence. However, justice has more to it than just fair distribution. For instance, vulnerable populations exploited for scientific research are entitled to compensation. That is to say, we have to deal sometimes with *rectificatory* justice, not only distribution. This is a limitation of Engelhardt's account of justice and shows that justice is not just an ingredient of beneficence.

A similar contractualistic approach to the foundations of bioethics, based on the priority of autonomy, was put forward by Robert M. Veath in his book *A Theory of Medical Ethics*. Veath considers his contract model a universal and objectivist attempt to determine ethical principles for medical ethics. Following the rehabilitation of the contract theory in ethics by John Rawls, his model comprises three contracts. The *first contract* is the most basic one and it specifies the content of the ethical system for all of society, based on the following principles: beneficence, autonomy,

---

[30] Tristram Engelhardt, *The Foundations of Bioethics*, (New York/Oxford: Oxford University Press, 1996), 121.
[31] Tristram Engelhardt, *The Foundations of Bioethics*, (New York/Oxford: Oxford University Press, 1996), 121.

honesty, avoidance of killing, justice and contract keeping.[32] It can be considered the basis of the common morality. The *second contract* exists between society and the different professional groups. It establishes role-specific duties, which arise not from within the professions, but from a social point of view.[33] In the *third contract*, particular questions of care are negotiated between health professionals and the patient. It establishes the boundaries of that relationship.[34] Many bioethicists follow a similar contractualist model, instead of a fiduciary one.

At this point, it is worth recalling the cases we are discussing to critically assess the autonomist view. In the Baby 1 story, according to Engelhardt's autonomist view, the parents have the last word: whatever they want should be provided. That is to say, he holds that we *must* respect the parents' wishes, choices, decisions etc. and increase care for Baby 1 no matter what. This is, however, unreasonable since it could produce more harm than good. In the Baby 2 case, some cultural differences between the two countries, the US and Brazil, would allow Engelhard to say that each should decide according to its values. But this is not consensual among bioethicists. For instance, in Pellegrino's view, doctors know better. Defending the model of "beneficence-in-trust", Pellegrino and Thomasma would not give too much weight to the parents' choices and would look for what the health team thinks is best for Baby 1 and Baby 2 from a caring point of view. We can also reach this conclusion by realizing that Pellegrino and Thomasma's main critique of autonomism is that it overemphasizes the right to self-determination but forgets the duty to restore and protect autonomy when it is absent. Let me then now contrast autonomism with this proposal, which prioritises beneficence over individual permission.

This renewed approach to bioethical problems came from a distinct philosophy of medicine *transforming* the Hippocratic tradition, recognising a place for autonomy while still stressing the priority of beneficence. Pellegrino and Thomasma argued that a new philosophy of medicine is needed in order to organize medicine's increasing number of successes, to form an integrating principle for its splintering specialties, to offer rational, scientific explanations of its methods, etc. Most importantly, a new philosophy of medicine is needed to help clarify medicine's goals in

[32] Robert Veath, *A Theory of Medical Ethics*, (New York: Basic Books, 1981), 110.
[33] Robert Veath, *A Theory of Medical Ethics*, (New York: Basic Books, 1981), 127f.
[34] Robert Veath, *A Theory of Medical Ethics*, (New York: Basic Books, 1981), 134f.

relation to those of a technological civilization, since medicine suffers from an abundance of means and a poverty of ends. Grounding medicine on an ontology of the body and seeing it as a value-laden practice, they first proposed three axioms: do no harm; respect the vulnerability of patients; treat all patients as equal members of the human race.[35] Basically, this means that the first and primary value is that it is good to be healthy and this is a basic need of living bodies, grounding the Hippocratic axiom. Moreover, the second principle presupposes that individuals have intrinsic value and thus care must be directed to the susceptible, the vulnerable individual. Finally, the intrinsic value of individuals includes their representation as a class-instance of human bodies (common to all living bodies) and this is the condition of possibility where cure takes place. Having established the framework of a professional ethics stemming from the axiom of vulnerability, the authors argued that primary care responds to such a human need and should therefore be universally accessible. This is not a political requirement, but supposedly a moral one springing from the goals of medicine itself.

The main question in assessing whether this model is acceptable is this: what constitutes the patient's good? According to Pellegrino and Thomasma, four main ingredients, *in descending order of importance*, are part of the patient's good. Briefly, they are:

i) the last or ultimate good, the *telos* of human life as it is perceived by the patient, his or her view of the meaning and destiny of human existence, the position taken with reference to relationships with other men and women, the world, and God;
ii) the good of the patient as a human person, the good that is grounded in his capacity as a human being to reason, and therefore to choose, and to express those choices in speech with other humans who can also reason and speak;
iii) the patient's best interests, that is, the patient's subjective assessment of the quality of life the intervention might produce, and whether or not he deems it consistent with his life plan, goals, and aims;

---

[35] Edmund Pellegrino and David Thomasma, *A Philosophical Basis of Medical Practice*, (New York/Oxford: Oxford University Press, 1981), 184f. For a general presentation of the beneficence-in-trust model in contrast to contractualist models, see chapter 4 of Pellegrino and Thomasma's book *For the Patient's Good.* For a comprehensive view of Pellegrinos's philosophy of medicine see: Tristram Engelhardt and Fabrice Jotterand (eds.), *The Philosophy of Medicine Reborn: a Pellegrino Reader*, (Notre Dame: University of Notre Dame Press, 2008).

iv) medical, biomedical, or clinical good –the good that can be achieved by medical interventions into a particular disease state.[36]

Note that even if Pellegrino and Thomasma argue for the primacy of beneficence, they allow for some ingredients (the first and third) of the patient's good to be based on her own views of what is valuable. But, ultimately, the patient's good is what benefits her regardless of what she prefers (the second and the last components). Thus, if this is true, then care would give us, so to speak, agent-neutral reasons for action. But the first element in their conception of the patient's good is, according to modern science, questionable for many reasons: there may be no *telos* for human life or intrinsic to medicine itself. There may be no ultimate good; it may be relative to a particular worldview only. Of course, it is a good thing to be healthy, but the place health occupies in one's life generates different axiological systems.

Pellegrino and Thomasma's main project, then, is to restore the prime place of beneficence in medicine, particularly in bioethics. They argue that the values of patients' welfare and patients' autonomy may be in conflict. To overcome this conflict, it is necessary to see the physician's end as healing, that is, a form of assistance in making the patient whole again by working on his or her body and mind.[37] This can be achieved by their beneficence-in-trust model. Leaving for now their criticism of the perils of autonomy aside, the basic norms of the beneficence-model they want to restore are the following points: (i) both doctor and patient must be free to make informed decisions and to act fully as moral agents; (ii) physicians have the greater responsibility in the relationship because of the inherent inequality of information and power between themselves and those who are ill; (iii) physicians must be persons of personal moral integrity; (iv) physicians must respect and comprehend moral ambiguity yet not abandon the search for what is right and good in each decision.[38]

---

[36] Edmund D. Pellegrino and David C. Thomasma, *For the Patient's Good*, (New York/Oxford: Oxford University Press, 1988), 81-2.

[37] In this sense, Pellegrino and Thomasma's conception of health is closer to the WHO's definition: "Health is a state of complete physical, mental and social wellbeing and not merely the absence of disease or infirmity." For a discussion on normative and descriptive conceptions of health see: Marco Antonio Azevedo's paper "Health as Clinic-Epidemiological Concept," *The Journal of Evaluation in Clinical Practice*, 21(3), 2015, 265f.

[38] Edmund D. Pellegrino and David C. Thomasma, *For the Patient's Good*, (New York/Oxford: Oxford University Press, 1988), 34-5.

It seems clear that Pellegrino and Thomasma think that respect for autonomy needs to be better balanced with beneficence, with a stronger compromise with care. The key to achieving that is to rethink beneficence not in the traditionally paternalistic terms but as based on *trust*. According to them,

> By beneficence-in-trust we mean that physicians and patients hold 'in trust' (Latin, *fiducia*) the goal of acting in the best interests of one another in the relationship. In the main, the patient's fulfilment of this trust resides in carrying out the negotiated plan for his or her health. The burden of trust more often belongs on the physician, who must act in the interests of the patient under the conditions we have already discussed, including social conditions.[39]

If physicians and patients are persons of moral integrity, they can trust each other. Onora O'Neill has also recently carried out a study from a Kantian point of view of the place of trust in special bioethics, including a critique of the ritual of informed consent as an expression of individual autonomy.[40] In fact, most health professionals do not care about informed consent, perhaps because they think that they must be trusted. In the Baby 2 case, the papers are there, but they are not signed. That is why O'Neill proposes to use a *Kantian* conception of autonomy to restore trust in bioethics as self-imposition of universal moral laws.

Pellegrino and Thomasma, however, have constantly criticized both autonomy and *strong* forms of paternalism (e.g., acting against someone's will) supposedly based on the Hippocratic tradition or on a utilitarian ethics, but yet are willing to restore beneficence in medicine as a prime value. They wrote:

> Medical paternalism fails because it overrides an essential element in deontological ethics at the core of medicine, that is, respect for persons. To violate the patient's autonomy is to deprive him or her of one essential component of her own good, and thus to violate medicine's promise to act for the good of the patient.[41]

---

[39] Edmund D. Pellegrino and David C. Thomasma, *For the Patient's Good*, (New York/Oxford: Oxford University Press, 1988), 54-5.

[40] Onora O'Neill, *Autonomy and Trust in Bioethics*, (Cambridge: Cambridge University Press, 2002). For a critical discussion of informed consent see also: Neil C. Manson and Onora O'Neill, *Rethinking Informed Consent in Bioethics*, (Cambridge: Cambridge University Press, 2007).

[41] Edmund D. Pellegrino and David C. Thomasma, *For the Patient's Good*, (New York/Oxford: Oxford University Press, 1988), 23.

The authors' primary aim is to argue for the good for the patient and that implies restoring the central place of beneficence in bioethics, without disrespecting patients' autonomy. It is doubtful, however, whether they can avoid *weak* or *soft* forms of paternalism, that is, acting *without* someone's consent in her benefit, but not necessarily against her will.

Actually, Pellegrino and Thomasma hold that no single principle of ethics could govern all health care practice, but at the same time they maintain that the value of beneficence is the more fundamental one. More accurately, they coined the expression 'beneficence-*in-trust*' to underline the fact that it encompasses beneficence with a concern for the patient's best interests including his autonomy. Thus, caring & respecting should go together according to the beneficence-in-trust model, but care still takes some priority and it seems to give agent-neutral reasons to act. As I have said, I will return to this point later when discussing Darwall's theory of rational care.

The beneficence-in-trust model is not, however, without critics. Beauchamp and Childress wrote on this proposal:

> Along these lines, two defenders of the beneficence model, Edmund Pellegrino and David Thomasma, argue that 'the best interest of the patients are intimately linked with their preferences,' from which 'are derived our primary duties toward them.' This formulation of the beneficence model simply restates the autonomy model. If the patient's preferences alone determine the content of the physician's obligation to act beneficently, respect for autonomy rather than pure medical beneficence has triumphed, and the problem of paternalism evaporates.[42]

This criticism seems not entirely fair. The beneficence-in-trust model relies on the Aristotelian idea of a virtuous physician's judgment about what is the good for the patient, whether she is autonomous or not.

The danger of paternalism remains. The beneficence-in-trust model assumes that there is an essential moral nature to medicine, which must guide professional practices. Granted: medicine is an *art*, which combines sciences and virtues. In the beneficence-in-trust model, if we pay attention to the list of the physician's virtues, for instance, *benevolence* and the patient's virtues, especially *trust*, we realize who is, so to speak, playing a passive and who is playing an active role. There is no doubt that this may lead to paternalism, even if it is in its soft or weak forms, that is,

[42] Tom L. Beauchamp and James F. Childress, *Principles of Biomedical Ethics*, (New York/Oxford: Oxford University Press, 2009), 207.

overriding one's choices but not necessarily against one's will. Consequently, we need a better balance between caring & respecting.

As we have seen, the Belmont Report gives equal weight to the basic principles, but we have now two opposite views: Engelhardt holds that the principle of autonomy is prior; Pellegrino and Thomasma maintain that beneficence has this status. In some medical headquarters, the beneficence model seems to be winning the debate. To recognize this point, it is worth mentioning another approach, similar to Pellegrino and Thomasma's model, which was put forward by the "Medical Professionalism in the New Millennium: a Physician Charter" issued by the American Board of Internal Medicine Foundation and the European Federation of Internal Medicine, signed in 2002. The charter requires physicians to follow these principles in *lexical order*:

i) patient welfare ("this principle is based on a dedication to serving the interest of the patient. Altruism contributes to the trust that is central to the physician-patient relationship. Market forces, societal pressures, and administrative exigencies must not compromise this principle.");
ii) patient autonomy ("physicians must have respect for patients' autonomy. Physicians must be honest with their patients and empower them to make informed decisions about their treatment. Patients decisions about their care must be paramount, as long as those decisions are in keeping with ethical practice and do not lead to demands for inappropriate care.");
iii) social justice ("The medical profession must promote justice in the health care system, including the fair distribution of health care resources. Physicians should work actively to eliminate discrimination in health care, whether based on race, gender, socioeconomic status, ethnicity, religion, or any other social category.")[43]

This inversion of priorities in relation to the autonomist view is, however, understandable since it represents the physician's point of view, which tends to be class-driven, but we need to remember that medicine is a practice which must be socially justified and legitimized. Its justification depends on the good that it is capable of providing, namely the prevention of illness and the maintenance of health and the effective cure of diseases. But, this may be *one* value among others in a person's axiological scale.

---

[43] http://www.ncbi.nlm.nih.gov/pubmed/11827500

As can be seen, the principle of beneficence, based on the Hippocratic Oath, took priority over autonomy in the physician's charter giving apparent victory to Pellegrino and Thomasma's arguments over Beauchamp and Childress's principlism and Engelhardt's autonomism. But critics complain that the traditional Hippocratic ethics is nowadays challenged by the introduction of tenets belonging to a modern view based on human individual rights. Thus, the debate between autonomists and defenders of the priority of beneficence still remains open.

At this juncture, one may wonder whether there is a way of overcoming the present "state of art" in bioethics, namely the divergent philosophical accounts of its normative foundations. Perhaps the long history of ethics, and the short life of bioethics, with the latter somehow reproducing the route of the former, is strong evidence, if not proof, of ethical relativism. In the next chapter, I will discuss the idea of *a* common morality as a way of avoiding relativism and providing stronger normative bases for bioethics.

CHAPTER FOUR

TOWARDS A COMMON, SHARABLE MORALITY

As I pointed out in the first chapter, despite the fact that caring & respecting can be regarded as two ways of intrinsically valuing an individual, they are subject to tensions, which generate apparent dilemmas and may even lead to inaction. We have also seen that there are different ways of recasting these tensions, and, in the previous two chapters, I reconstructed some discussions on the normative foundations of bioethics as an illustration of this difficulty. Thus, the theoretical differences between the principles of the Belmont Report (based on the three *prima facie* norms of respect for persons, beneficence and justice), the principlists (based on the four principles of respect for autonomy, non-maleficence, beneficence and justice), the autonomists (who prioritize the principle of individual permission over beneficence and justice to avoid dilemmas) and the model of beneficence-in-trust (prioritizing the principle of the Hippocratic tradition instead) are examples of an ongoing debate with divergent practical implications. Now, recalling Lantos' characterization of the development of neonatal bioethics, he argued that doctors didn't *know how*, for instance, to apply the Baby Doe guidelines. Thus, it seems that we need in fact a *new moral epistemology* to solve these problems working more closely with the notions of *caring*, which seems to include both non-maleficence and beneficence, and *respecting*, which incorporates the rights to self-determination, to fair distribution etc. Before elaborating this new epistemology, we need then to re-analyse both care & respect and this will be done in this chapter. Afterwards, I will try to find a way of integrating them into a coherent moral system based on a solid normative ethics and that will be done in the next chapter. I will then argue that we need to ground a common moral system on a new moral epistemology. There I will sort out the concept of respectful care, based on practical cognitivism, that is, on the idea that moral knowledge is best understood as involving knowing-how. This new epistemology must be capable of solving the tensions in the meta-ethical and normative bases of bioethics. In the following chapters, I will apply the concept of respectful care, illustrating how it can work in practice.

4.1 Re-analysing care & respect

The common confusions regarding the meta-ethical and normative bases of bioethics may have as their main cause a misunderstanding concerning the moral nature of caring & respecting. In this section, then, I will rediscuss the ways they conflict and how we can solve them. To achieve this aim, I will re-analyse both concepts *reducing* the four principles of bioethics to these two notions. Moreover, I will start to examine the idea of *a* common, sharable morality as based on a single attitude, namely respectful care, as a way of integrating the two basic moral attitudes in the foundations of bioethics. It will be crucial to understand the correct meta-ethical characterization of reasons to care & reasons to respect. Clarifying the nature of these reasons for action is also an important aim of the present section.

Before attempting a reduction of the four principles approach to the concepts of care & respect, let me point out that another important change in the book *Principles of Biomedical Ethics* was the introduction of the idea of *the* common morality. In fact, this idea was best defended by Gert, Culver and Clouser in their book *Bioethics: a Return to Fundamentals* and was later incorporated by the principlists. Thus, according to Beauchamp and Childress, the assumption is that "the common morality is not merely *a* morality, in contrast to other moralities; it is *the* morality."[1] I will critically discuss this idea. As we will see, one difference between my proposal and common morality theories is that one must consider a common system comprising mutual caring and reciprocal respectful attitudes to be *a* morality among others, but not *the* morality despite the fact that it plays a special role in a pluralist society. Thus, my proposal of *a* common, *sharable* morality, which will be sorted out from now on, is not conceived in terms of *the* absolute morality, a-historical, a-social, immutable, etc.

To show why it is doubtful whether we can assume the existence of this kind of moral system (the true and eternal one), let me briefly comment on Gert, Culver and Clouser's argument for the existence of *the* common morality. They wrote: "Common morality is the foundation on which we build: first by explicating how morality works, then by justifying the practice as a public system for everyone, and finally by showing how it is manifested in different cultures, including subcultures

---

[1] Tom L. Beauchamp and James F. Childress, *Principles of Biomedical Ethics*, (New York/Oxford: Oxford University Press, 2013), 3.

like professions, all the while remaining one integrated morality."[2] Their approach to morality is grounded on "certain universal features of humankind" and it is mainly specified in ten rules such as "don't deceive," "don't kill," "keep your promises," "obey the law" etc.[3] The main philosophical problem with Gert, Culver and Clouser's argument for *the* common morality is that they grounded it on a moral theory that relies ultimately on *intuitions*,[4] which is a fuzzy foundation indeed: my intuition tells me this (e.g., disobey the law whenever it is unfair and therefore not legitimate), while yours may tell you otherwise (that is, always obey this law even if it is unjust). More importantly, the moral life cannot be reduced to following rules. Ethics needs a better phenomenology of the moral life, describing the role of sentiments, institutions, rules, emotions, principles, values, ideals etc. Unfortunately, to develop this point goes beyond the scope of this work, but some elements of caring & respecting such as sympathy and rights will become apparent soon, since they are the main components of *a* common, sharable morality. I will return to Gert, Culver and Clouser's proposal of the common morality later in this chapter while discussing the differences between *killing* and *letting die*. For now, let us speak in more modest terms of *a* morality, not *the* morality, the eternal and immutable one.

It seems clear that we live in an age of moral uncertainty. The stories of Baby 1 and Baby 2 need not be transformed into paradigmatic cases, but they clearly reveal that the conflicts between caring & respecting are still going on even after almost forty years of bioethical regulations, and that they have not come to a satisfactory solution yet. In the case of Baby 1, both parties seem to have made mistakes: on the one hand, the parents apparently didn't *know how* to stop even when only harm could come to their daughter by continuing treatment, and in this way they were not providing the best possible care for *her*; the parents seemingly disrespected the health team calling one member "the almost doctor" or "the pretend doctor in training" and saying that the nurses were "pretending to care for their daughter"; on the other hand, the health team apparently disrespected the parents by not taking seriously the conditions of "informed consent" such as using clear language in the disclosure of Baby 1's diagnosis and prognosis leading to a misunderstanding about

---

2 Bernard Gert and Charles Culver and Danner Clouser, *Bioethics*, (New York/Oxford: Oxford University Press, 1997), 1.

3 Bernard Gert and Charles Culver and Danner Clouser, *Bioethics*, (New York/Oxford: Oxford University Press, 1997), 34.

4 Bernard Gert and Charles Culver and Danner Clouser, *Bioethics*, (New York/Oxford: Oxford University Press, 1997), 3.

what "palliative care" would amount to in these circumstances; they apparently disrespected the parents by taking away their right to decide what was best for the baby; the Ethics Committee apparently disrespected Baby 1 by not giving her another chance to live when she was not allowed to be transferred and get a *real* second opinion; the Legal System seems to have disrespected the parents' wishes by not immediately giving them a "restraining order"; the Media apparently disrespected everyone by playing a power game in a case where a cool decision was necessary. That is to say, caring & respecting were almost ignored and that may have cost Baby 1's life. In the Baby 2 case, there were also rights and wrongs in the caring process but, overall, saving her was the best decision despite the fact that she now has less quality of life than can be expected for a person without disabilities. I will return to these cases in chapter 6 saying in a more conclusive way what was right or wrong after re-analysing care & respect and after making explicit how *practical cognitivism* grounds *respectful care* for *a common, sharable morality*.

How can we best deal with these conflicts in order to avoid them happening again? To answer this question, we need to scrutinize further the sources of these clashes and have a better understanding of what is required to integrate care & respect into a coherent moral life. One way of explaining the tensions is to look more closely at the supposed antagonism between two conceptions of morality. Briefly speaking, the predominant tradition in Western medicine, from the classical era, based on the Hippocratic Oath, which became official in the Middle Ages in Europe, was guided by the beneficence ideal, which basically meant caring for the patient, including curing her when that was possible. Now, this tradition takes the good of the patient, understood basically in terms of her health as central to her wellbeing as the aim of medical practice. Pellegrino's model, as we saw in the last chapter, follows this ideal. This tradition was dominant until modernity questioned the idea of the *Summum Bonum* and replaced it with the individual's right to choose what kind of life she wants to live and the place of health within it. This individual right to freedom as well as the rights to property and the pursuit of happiness were at the centre of the Modern Revolutions (English, American, French, etc.) and reshaped not only the political scenario, forging a new vision of the state based on *a hypothetical contract* among citizens, but also all the domains of social and public life such as law, medicine etc. Since the physician and philosopher John Locke, who had a great influence on the writing of the US Constitution and, consequently, on the creation of North-American values, placed *individual* rights before the state's policies, respect for a person's choices came to be even more important than the traditional values of the good life. In Locke's terms: "The *State of Nature* has a Law of Nature to govern it, which obliges every one: And Reason, which is that Law, teaches all Mankind, who will but consult it, that being all equal and independent, no one ought to harm another in his Life, Health, Liberty, or Possessions."[5] Note that among rights is health, not only liberty and property. This ideal was somehow carried on by the civil rights movement in the 1960s in the US leading to the formation of the National Commission to examine the Tuskegee case, which resulted in the Belmont Report analysed previously. Thus, the conflicts between caring & respecting may reflect the clash of the traditional approach to medicine with the modern view about its role within a pluralistic society. Traditionally, caring was the very purpose of medicine and respect for the patient's will was almost absent; modernity reversed that: respect for the patient's autonomy came to be, at least, as equal as –if not more important– than caring. What we need then is to reconcile care & respect into a single morality, *a* common and sharable one, based on *respectful care*.

Another way of understanding the tensions between caring & respecting is to recognize the conflicts in the *ethical theories* themselves. In the past years, different forms of ethical particularism, including *ethics of care* (and narrative ethics, virtue ethics, feminist ethics etc.) have held that it is necessary to consider the medical history of the patient, the particular circumstances of her life within her family, the details of *her* healing conditions, etc... In this way, caring, especially in the context of clinical treatment (either direct/acute or indirect/chronic, intensive or palliative etc.), involves taking a look at the singularities of the individual patient. Thus, caring could be seen as essentially related to a feminine/feminist approach to morality, while respect for persons would be based on rights and impartial, universal principles of justice, a typical "male" approach. This seems, however, to be a misunderstanding since Gilligan argues that an ethics of responsibility and an ethics of rights actually complement each other. To recognize this point, it is sufficient to re-read the epigraph of this work. Moreover, if we consider an ethics of care as a variation of an ethics of virtue and attempt to overcome the division between consequentialists, deontologists and virtue ethicists, then we will not have *philosophical* reasons to oppose care & respect. In the next chapter, I will amend Parfit's Triple Theory in order to overcome these main divisions in normative ethics.

[5] John Locke, *Two Treatises of Government,* (Cambridge: Cambridge University Press, 1994), 271).

Another possible source of conflict between caring & respecting may be found in an upside-down meta-ethical characterization of the kind of reasons for action each one generates. To use Darwall's way of putting it: "Reasons for acting that are rooted in respect are *second-personal, agent-regarding, and agent-relative.* ... Reasons of care, on the other hand, are *third-personal, welfare-regarding,* and *agent-neutral.*"[6] At first sight, however, it seems that the very opposite is the case: care seems to generate agent-relative reasons for actions, and respect, agent-neutral. That is to say, it looks like I may have strong reasons to care for my little daughter, but not for the strangers living on the other side of the planet; equally, I must respect an unknown person, indeed any stranger around me. Now, one could think that if reasons to care are regarded as agent-neutral and to respect as agent-relative, and if agent-neutral reasons trump relative ones, then care may degenerate into paternalism potentially leading to disrespect. That is why we need to re-examine some of Darwall's characterizations of the meta-ethical features of caring & respecting to avoid paternalism and, most importantly, to clarify what it means to say that a reason to act is either agent-neutral or agent-relative.[7]

One of the main present-day challenges in bioethics is harmoniously to integrate care & respect into a coherent whole for our moral life. As we have seen, these two main bioethical notions may not always be internally linked and can even be in conflict. In fact, care & respect relate to two different moral attitudes. If one cares for an individual, that is, if one is concerned with her welfare, it should matter what happens to her wellbeing. This may not be the case with respect: one may respect a person, to use Kant's words, never treating her as a mere means, never abusing her in any form (emotional, physical, economic etc.) even if apparently one does not care about what happens to her in various domains of her life. As Kant puts it, the principle of respect requires that two persons "keep themselves *at a distance* from one another."[8] For instance, I may walk around the campus "giving respect and expecting it" without doing any possible good, so to speak, to the strangers around me. In other

[6] Stephen Darwall, *Welfare and Rational Care*, (Princeton/Oxford: Princeton University Press, 2004), 127.

[7] For a criticism of this distinction see: Christine M. Korsgaard, "The Reasons We Can Share. An Attack on the Distinction between Agent-Relative and Agent-Neutral Value" (*Social Philosophy and Policy*, 1993, 10(1)). But Korsgaard, in fact, conflates these notions (e.g., agent-relative with subjective) and my distinction between two senses of 'agent-neutral' aims at avoiding this confusion.

[8] Immanuel Kant, *The Metaphysics of Morals*, (Cambridge: Cambridge University Press, 1996), 569 (6: 449).

words, respect may be a *negative* attitude only. Therefore, it looks like care requires both the principles of non-maleficence and beneficence; respect, only the former.

There seems to be a *limit* that respect imposes on caring. To illustrate: a father caring too much for his grown up son, his concern taking even an anxious form, may lead to paternalistic actions or attitudes, which are certainly a form of disrespect. When your son was a child, care perhaps was all he needed. Now, education requires him to respect you as a father and here respect means only: he has to recognize your authority as the one caring. But this is not the only meaning of 'respect,' and now that he is an adult person, mutual respect is required. Thus, as Darwall pointed out, we must distinguish between *appraisal* and *recognition* respect.[9] The former involves admiration for one's acts; the second relates to personhood itself. Thus, a central question is this: how to really respect someone in the latter sense? Is respect just obedience to a higher ranking individual's role (the father/son case) or is it due to all persons in the sense of a deference to their rights? A plausible answer seems to be that respect is due to all persons equally generating then agent-neutral reasons to act also, but before assuming that this is the case, it is necessary to re-analyse the concept of respect to identify its proper object and the relevant attitude it requires. The same applies to care: we need to identify its proper object and the other ingredients it is composed of.

In order to re-analyse care & respect, I will rely on Darwall's rational theory of welfare (henceforth, RTW). Thus, I will reconstruct now some of his ideas. In his book *Welfare and Rational Care,* he offers one of the most interesting recent theories about care, closely connected with the need to respect persons. Darwall holds that caring for someone *is* wanting her welfare for *her* own sake and that "… a person's good is constituted, not by what that person values, prefers, or wants (or should value), but by what one (perhaps she) should want *insofar as one cares about her*."[10] Thus, a person's welfare constitutes what benefits *her*, not necessarily what she actually prefers, but what she *ought to* desire from a *rational* perspective, that is, from the perspective of a person *caring* for her. This is the core idea of the rational theory of welfare. The central idea of this theory is that the good of a person, in the sense of what benefits *her*, may differ from what she herself values, prefers, or takes interest in at a given moment. To relate this theory to our previous discussions on the

[9] Stephen Darwall, *The Second-Person Standpoint*, (Cambridge/London: Harvard University Press, 2006), 122-6.

[10] Stephen Darwall, *Welfare and Rational Care*, (Princeton/Oxford: Princeton University Press, 2004), 4.

foundations of bioethics, it has more affinity with Pellegrino's beneficence-in-trust model rather than the preferentialist or autonomist views such as the one held by Engelhardt. A concern relating to the RTW, however, is whether it does not lead also to some forms of paternalism, producing an unbalanced relation between caring & respecting.

Despite the fact that Darwall's account of welfare's normativity has much to recommend it, especially the way he links care with psychological states such as sympathy, empathy etc., his meta-ethical characterization of care as agent-neutral deserves to be re-examined. I believe saying that reasons to care *simpliciter* are agent-neutral (and respect, agent-relative) may be misleading since such an account of *rational* care may be in danger of paternalism. For instance, an autocratic doctor could say "I am *the one caring* here, so do as I say. I know what is best for your welfare!" actually disrespecting a patient. This was the traditional Hippocratic approach. That is to say, it may lead to overriding the subject/patient's own beliefs, values and, most importantly, her rights. This would be disrespectful indeed. Thus, we have to find a way of avoiding such a negative consequence by *limiting* care with recognition respect, a point that is not always clear in the RTW. This theory, when linked to the "Aristotelian Thesis," namely the idea that the most beneficial human life consists of activities involving the appreciation of worth and merit, especially a virtuous life, may have doubtful applications in our bioethical cases since it may perhaps lead to paternalist actions. In Darwall's own words, "the Aristotelian Thesis asserts that a life of virtuous activity is best *for the person herself*, what benefits *her* most."[11] Despite the fact that I think that his Aristotelian thesis may only be partially true (we cannot link a premature baby's welfare to it), I would like to point out that my conceptual analysis of *respectful care*, which will be presented in the next chapter, was greatly inspired by Darwall's own account, yet I will try to avoid the apparent paternalistic implications of regarding care as agent-neutral in an unqualified way.

To achieve this aim, I would like to add a few critical comments on Darwall's Aristotelian thesis. He holds that a life of virtuous activity is best *for the person herself*, what benefits *her* most.[12] Let us, however, ask in the case of a premature baby: what could a life of virtuous activity possibly be? Indeed, a baby's wellbeing may be seen as giving agent-neutral reasons to act, but it cannot relate to a virtuous life or any other

---

[11] Stephen Darwall, *Welfare and Rational Care*, (Princeton/Oxford: Princeton University Press, 2004), 82.

[12] Stephen Darwall, *Welfare and Rational Care*, (Princeton/Oxford: Princeton University Press, 2004), 82.

activity involving the appreciation of worth and merit. That is to say, this applies to adults only. A baby's welfare must be constituted by something else, for instance, absence of pain and suffering, adequate nutrition, healthy intestines etc. In other words, by satisfying her basic needs. Thus, it is right to say "welfare's normativity is not agent-relative; it is agent-neutral," but there is a sense in which welfare's normativity needs to be seen as agent-relative too. We need to build up a common, sharable morality where care & respect are integrated into a coherent whole in the right balanced way to avoid this problem.

It is worth discussing further whether Darwall's RTW is really capable of avoiding *strong* forms of paternalism. To have a clear understanding of this point, it is important to point out that Darwall also considers reasons for action rooted in respect to be *agent-regarding*. That is to say, respect for persons is "a responsiveness to what makes them persons, the capacity for free agency. What we must attend to here is not, primarily anyway, what is for someone's good, but what she holds good and would want from her point of view."[13] For instance, it makes perfect sense to make one's child eat her broccoli, but once she is a young adult person it would be considered paternalistic to exert undue pressure to make her abandon unhealthy habits and to keep eating broccoli. Thus, respect for persons, given that reasons to respect are agent-regarding too, may block paternalistic actions based on partial interpretations of the RTW. I will, however, argue that considering *recognition respect* as giving *agent-neutral reasons* to act seems to be a better way of envisaging how to avoid strong forms of paternalism, that is, when care could lead to disrespectful actions. This is the path I will follow to try to integrate care & respect.

There is a sense, I believe, that reasons to care are agent-relative and reasons to respect are agent-neutral. To recognize this point, let me recall the case of Baby 1. There are reasons to care for the baby that are, in a specific sense (let us call this meaning "*in the non-positional sense*"), agent-neutral. That is to say, *anyone* has, on the one hand, a reason to hold that children must be properly cared for, that is, they must receive the medical attention they have a right to. I think that this is the case with Baby 1 as it must be with any baby indeed. This shows that any form of particularism in bioethics is misconceived. Of course, we should pay close attention to all the relevant features of particular cases, but since reasons for caring are agent-neutral in the non-positional sense, it follows that the same holds for every other case, namely Baby 1, Baby 2, Baby 3 (who will

---

[13] Stephen Darwall, *Welfare and Rational Care*, (Princeton/Oxford: Princeton University Press, 2004), 15.

be presented in the next chapter) … and Baby X. That children do not starve, that children are properly cared for by their own parents, that children receive the medical attention they need from health professionals is an agent-neutral reason for action, that is, it is an impartial and universal one. Therefore, an ethics of care need not be particularist. On the other hand, Baby 1's parents have agent-relative reasons, *in the positional sense* (that is, referring to them as agents, but not depending necessarily on their preferences and desires), to care for *their* own child that other agents do not necessarily have. Moreover, health caregivers at the U. of A. also have agent-relative reasons to care for their patients, especially for Baby 1, which other people do not have. I cannot possibly have an agent-relative reason in this sense to care for an extremely premature baby since I do not know how to prescribe parenteral nutrition. That does not mean that they have *subjective* reasons for caring for the patient as they like. That is to say, agent-relativity in this case means only that these professionals have *special obligations* to care for a vulnerable being, their patient. General care may be an imperfect duty, but *special* care, for parents and health care professionals, is a strict and perfect obligation.

Having re-examined the meta-ethical nature of reasons to care & reasons to respect and made the distinction between the positional and non-positional sense, it is time now to present a conceptual analysis of both care & respect. As I said above, I will rely on Darwall's RTW despite the fact that I have partially rejected his Aristotelian thesis and clarified further the meta-ethical characterization of reasons to care & reasons to respect saying in which sense they are either agent-neutral or agent-relative. Thus, let me first ask under which necessary and sufficient conditions we may say that a person cares for a vulnerable being. Recalling Nodding's analytical model presented in the introduction and using the RTW, we may say that the following situation (W, X) is a caring relation iff:

i) W sympathizes with X;
ii) X's welfare needs attention;
iii) W benefits X for *her* own sake.

I hope these are the necessary and sufficient conditions to apply the concept of 'care' in special bioethical contexts. Of course, there may be other contexts where 'care' means something different, for instance, when we say that one takes care of a particular pen. We must, therefore, keep in mind the special bioethical context while applying this concept. It provides an alternative to Nodding's analysis since her model presents conditions that are not necessary (e.g., recognition) and conjointly are not sufficient. My analysis leads to the following definition of 'special care': benefitting out of sympathy someone's welfare for her own sake. It reveals that care is a way of intrinsically valuing a vulnerable being. An apparent limitation of this analysis is, however, that it does not explicitly guarantee *respectful* actions.

To avoid misunderstandings, it is worth pointing out that I am not searching for *analytic* definitions of the basic bioethical concepts. As Nick Zangwill has correctly pointed out against analytic moral functionalist views, it is doubtful whether substantial moral notions work in that way.[14] As I have argued elsewhere (2000), Moore's attempts to ground ideal utilitarianism in analytic definitions (e.g., of 'right') are doomed to failure. A definition gives only a rule to use a concept. In this sense, it is in some sense both "analytic" and "synthetic" at the same time. This is a way of avoiding the paradox of analysis and, consequently, the above model is not jeopardized by this problem.

A similar analytical model may then be presented to clarify the nature of 'respect'. Thus, let us ask under which necessary and sufficient conditions a person respects another person. Recalling Darwall's distinctions between kinds of respect, we may say that W respects X iff:

i) W recognizes X as a person (p);
ii) p has rights and/or obligations;
iii) W fulfils her obligations towards X for *her* own sake.

These are the necessary and I hope sufficient conditions to apply the concept of 'respect'. Again, there are different senses of 'respect' and we must bear in mind the special context we are working on. It leads to the definition of respect as the recognition of a person's rights and the fulfilment of the correspondent obligations for the person's own sake.

Now, in the non-positional sense, it becomes clear from the above analysis that recognition respect gives us agent-neutral reasons to act too. Moreover, the analytical model reveals that respect is also an intrinsic valuation of the person. There is no need to claim to have presented the final analysis of care & respect since some *ingredients* may be subject to further analyses in searching for the elements. An important and provisional result, however, is the definitions specifying the rules to apply these concepts in special bioethical contexts.

---

[14] Nick Zangwill, "Against Analytic Moral Functionalism," (*Ratio*. XIII, 3, 2000), 275f. See also Richard Hare's *Sorting Out Ethics*, (Oxford: Clarendon Press, 2000) for a similar point.

A further theoretical development would be to show that the principles of non-maleficence and beneficence can be *reduced* to care and that the principles of respect for autonomy (individual self-determination) and the principles of distributive justice can be *reduced* to respect. Clearly, this is the case because respect for persons includes both rights, namely self-determination and fair share in the distribution of a good, and many others indeed. Thus, the principle of respect for persons has more extension than respect for autonomy only. I will examine whether care can be reduced to respect or the other way around later. Before attempting to do that, we need to discuss whether care & respect can be integrated into the concept of *respectful care*. In order to do so, we may use the above analytical models. The concept of respectful care has the potential to overcome the meta-ethical and normative problems at the foundations of bioethics. I will present a conceptual analysis of respectful care in the next chapter.

At this juncture, one may wonder whether maintaining that we have agent-neutral reasons to care provides a sound justification for the *obligation* to benefit an individual's wellbeing for *her* own sake. Now, for those not convinced yet, I will try to arrive at the same result from a different angle. I would like to reconstruct now one of the most recent attempts to ground the obligation to care from an ethics of care perspective. Thus, let me put in the canonical format what can be called "The Obligation to Care Argument" sorted out by Daniel Engster (italics in the original):[15]

> Premise 1*: all human beings can be assumed to value their survival, the development and functioning of their basic capabilities, and the avoidance or alleviation of unwanted pain and suffering, unless they explicitly indicate otherwise;*
>
> Premise 2*: all human beings depend upon the care of others to survive, develop and maintain their basic capabilities, and avoid or alleviate unwanted pain and suffering;*
>
> Premise 3*: all human beings can be said at least implicitly to value caring as a necessary good and to make claims on others for care when we need it, meaning that we at least implicitly assert that others should help us to meet our basic needs, develop and maintain our basic capabilities, and avoid or alleviate pain when we cannot reasonably achieve these goods on our own;*
>
> Premise 4*: in claiming care from others, we imply that capable human beings ought to help individuals in need when they are able to do so consistent with their other caring obligations;*

[15] Daniel Engster, *The Heart of Justice*, (Oxford: Oxford University Press, 2011), 46-48.

Premise 5: *since all human beings depend upon the care of others for our survival, development, and basic functioning and at least implicitly claim that capable individuals should care for individuals in need when they can do so, we should consistently recognize as morally valid the claim that others make upon us for care when they need it, and should endeavor to provide care to them when we are capable of doing so without significant danger to ourselves, seriously compromising our long-term functioning, or undermining out ability to care for others.*

Conclusion ("the upshot of this argument"): "All individuals have a right to care."[16]

If we now ask whether this argument is valid (the conclusion really follows from the premises) and correct (all the premises are true), the answer must take into account that Engster started to justify the *obligation* to care, but arrived at a *right* to care. That is to say, the interconnections of this "dialectically necessary method" are not clear, despite the fact that I believe the premises are self-evident. Therefore, I will reform the argument stating a different conclusion, namely that we all have the obligation to care as it was above defined.

This is not, however, the only problem in Engster's account of care ethics, which may be adjusted anyway. If the results of the present section are sound, namely that care & respect are complementary, but yet *limit* each other, Engster cannot consider respect *a virtue* to be inferred from care.[17] In fact, if he wants to make sense of his own claim that "Individuals do always have the right to refuse the care of others,"[18] then we need a stronger notion of respect based on an equal recognition of persons and not just an appreciation of others' needs. A right to refuse care cannot be grounded in care itself, only on respect for persons. This shows also that neither respect can be reduced to care nor care to respect, without substantial loss. It is crucial to bear in mind that they *limit* each other avoiding both indifference and paternalism.

Apart from the self-evident *agent-neutral* character of reasons based on care (in the non-positional sense) and the cogency of the *obligation* to care argument, I will from now on assume that there is *a right* to be cared for (and a correspondent obligation from others to care) based on a personhood

---

[16] Daniel Engster, *The Heart of Justice*, (Oxford: Oxford University Press, 2011), 53.

[17] Daniel Engster, *The Heart of Justice*, (Oxford: Oxford University Press, 2011), 31.

[18] Daniel Engster, *The Heart of Justice*, (Oxford: Oxford University Press, 2011), 47.

account of human rights.[19] This right has already appeared when I quoted Locke previously. Now, briefly speaking, this account of rights states that a right to be cared for (together with the right to liberties and forms of equality and equity) is an intrinsic protection of normative agency itself for any member of our lifeform. It is therefore constitutive of personhood itself. If so, it is an *entitlement*, not merely a *claim* right. That is to say, it is an intrinsic right of personhood itself and not a contingent right, for instance, that a parent has at a given moment. That is why the principle of respect for persons remains central in special bioethics, and it is a cornerstone of *a* common, sharable morality. I will return to *respect for persons* in chapter 6.

If we accept that there is a right to be cared for, the immediate question is "whose duties?" In this sense, I believe that Engster has not only identified distinct ways of caring for others (personally or by providing caregivers with resources or collectively supporting institutions and policies that directly help individuals to meet their basic needs), but has also formulated an interesting political theory for a *caring* government worth discussing further.[20] I will here follow his design for the basic institutions of a caring government. Central to this institutional arrangement is certainly a fair health system. In this sense, we may just remember Beauchamp and Childress' proposal for a mixed system presented in the previous chapter. It may be justified by the principle of distributive justice now reduced to respect for persons, and it provides a model to rethink different existing systems, both the North American and the Brazilian/British ones.

Having hopefully identified some sources of the misunderstandings that lead to dilemmas, and having presented an analysis of both care & respect and reproduced a justification to the right to be cared for, let me now go back to the idea of the common morality and say a few more words about why we need to assume *a* common, sharable morality and not subscribe to *the* common one as Gert, Culver and Clouser and later Beauchamp and Childress did. My main reason to doubt their conception of *the* moral system comes from their particular solutions to the euthanasia and assisted suicide issues discussed in the last chapter of the book *Bioethics: a Return to Fundamentals*. After rejecting the basic criteria

---

[19] For a similar justification of a human right to welfare (the object of caring) see James Griffin, *On Human Rights*, (Oxford: Oxford University Press, 2013), 179f. For a critical assessment of Griffin's account see Roger Crisp, *Griffin on Human Rights*, (Oxford: Oxford University Press, 2014).

[20] Daniel Engster, *The Heart of Justice*, (Oxford: Oxford University Press, 2011), 31

normally used to distinguish active from passive euthanasia (act/omission, stopping/non-starting treatment, ordinary/extraordinary care, natural/non-natural death), the authors of *Bioethics* argued that if we use instead the difference between *patient request* and *patient refusal*, we will recognize that doctors must never kill, thus active euthanasia is always out of the question, but passive euthanasia or assisted dying (not suicide, but palliative care instead) is not only morally permissible, but *morally required*.[21] This "solution" puts all the responsibility on the patients' choices in order to maintain the doctors' social image, that is, they do not want to be seen as people prepared to kill, even mercifully. This presupposes an intrinsic *telos* to medicine that can no longer be sustained. Thus, in the case of Baby 1, there is no plausible reason to say that the terminally ill patient should not have been killed but only allowed to die. Many bioethicists have argued that letting die is, if there is any significant distinction here, worse than killing. We should then recognize the *social* nature of medicine and that its ends are established by our common interests, among them the option of a quick death if desired by a patient in such a condition or by her parents, without endorsing extreme forms of relativism. I will develop this argument in the next section preparing the path for the idea of *a* common, sharable morality based on practical cognitivism. Thus, I will question Gert, Culver and Clouser's reasons for holding that "When there is no medical treatment which is keeping the patient alive, stopping food and fluids may sometimes be the only way of allowing a patient to die."[22] The issue of killing or letting die provides us with a test of what must belong to the jurisdiction of *a* common, *sharable* morality and what must remain in the domain of particular moralities.

4.2 End-of-life care: killing or letting die?

Having pointed out that both care & *recognition* respect give us agent-neutral reasons to act, I would now like to discuss in more detail what care requires, for instance, at the end of life. This will be a way of testing the previous analysis of 'special care'. What does caring for the vulnerable really imply, for instance, in the Baby 1 case when treatment is futile, that is, a cure is not possible? Is palliative care always the best option or is active non-voluntary euthanasia morally permissible as an expression of

---

[21] Bernard Gert and Charles Culver and Danner Clouser, *Bioethics*, (New York/Oxford: Oxford University Press, 1997), 269-310.

[22] Bernard Gert and Charles Culver and Danner Clouser, *Bioethics*, (New York/Oxford: Oxford University Press, 1997), 292.

compassionate care? In this section, I will start to provide an answer to these questions considering the results of the present work so far. I will do so by examining in a more detailed way what should have been done in the case of Baby 1. This story will guide us in the direction of some bioethical conclusions. I will return to this and the other cases after presenting the concept of *respectful care*, that is, I will say in a more conclusive way in chapter 6 what should have been done in the Baby 1 case.

Let me then briefly recall some of the facts of Baby 1's story. A special kind of care, namely "palliative" care was offered to the parents after NEC was diagnosed and no available treatment was recommended by the health team at the U. of A. It seems clear, however, that the juridical battle between the medical team and the parents would not have existed if the latter had really understood and effectively agreed on the best end-of-life caring process. Did the parents' *consent* to *palliative* care at some point? How? There is no written directive allowing "palliative" care, that is, giving permission to discontinue life support.

At this juncture, it is crucial to be crystal clear on the conditions of consent. Bioethicists normally establish the following ones: i) competence to understand and decide; ii) voluntariness iii) disclosure; iv) recommendation of a plan; v) understanding; vi) decision in favour of a plan; and finally (vii) authorization of the chosen plan.[23] Thus, informed consent is one of the most important applications of the principle of respect for persons, specifying the right to self-determination. In the case of Baby 1, it seems clear that having the competence to understand is essential, but also, equally, is the *disclosure* of information. Thus, the civil litigation was perhaps caused by the health team's failure to reveal in *clear* language the kind of care they were recommending for the baby and the consequences of such a course of action.

According to the family's blog, these were the options given to them:

> 1: Do nothing and let her body start shutting down on its own;
> 2: Let us hold her while they begin turning equipment off;
> 3: Say good bye and walk away then have them turn life support off.

There is no doubt that the health team should have explained in a clearer way to the family, as reasonable persons, what, in fact, they really

---

[23] For an explanation of these conditions see: Tom Beauchamp and James Childress, *Principles of Biomedical Ethics*, (New York/Oxford: Oxford University Press, 2013), 124f. This seems to be another fine example of sorting out the necessary and *sufficient* conditions for informed consent carried out by Beauchamp and Childress.

were going to do. It seems clear that the parents were competent, that they were not forced (they were acting voluntarily), that the disclosure in fact was made, that a plan was presented to the family, *but* there are real doubts whether the family *understood* what *palliative* or *comfort* care means. Can anyone understand the first alternative "do nothing" as implying withdrawal of nutrition?

Astonishingly enough, this was even presented as a defendant's answer in court:

> As the best defendants can gather from the remaining allegations, Mr. and Mrs. XYZ *seem to be confusing* comfort care (giving optimal pain care through medications (morphine in this case), easing the work of breathing by optimizing ventilator settings and oxygen intake, and making the patient as comfortable as possible) with medical treatment (using intravenous tubes to give blood or blood components, antibiotics, and nutrition) that is of no benefit to Baby 1: she receives mechanical ventilatory support to that she can breathe (italics added).[24]

There are no excuses: it is a health team's *obligation*, a social worker's task perhaps, to present in clear language the options available so that the parents can exercise their right to decide. At this point, the medical team simply cannot defend themselves by saying that the parents do not understand the difference between *caring for* and *treatment* providing cure. As seems clear from the family's blog, this condition was not met and, therefore, the health team at the U. of A. seems to have made a serious mistake here. If so, this was *disrespectful* indeed. The patient has a right to information, not only to be cared for. One may, then, conclude that the alleged order validity, which the defendants argued "was still in effect"[25] at that moment seems invalid since the parents in fact did not understand what comfort care really implied for their daughter.

At this point, it may be helpful to present a clear definition of *palliative* care. There is no doubt that it is the product of a special knowledge to benefit helplessly suffering patients if and only if treatment is futile. Thus, palliative care means removing as much suffering as possible once a cure is no longer available. Palliative care, however, does not necessarily imply either active or passive euthanasia. But, in the Baby 1 case, it meant passive euthanasia, although this was not really said to the parents, withdrawing medical treatment including nutrition. Palliative care could in the Baby 1 case include keeping nutrition. The crucial question then is

---

[24] Case No. 06 1015 CZ, Answer to complaint, p.16-7.

[25] Case No. 06 1015 CZ, Answer to complaint, 9.

whether food is a kind of treatment. It is argued that, if nutrition is a treatment prescribed by the medical team, it can be withdrawn and it is not part of palliative care. However, some bioethicists have argued that feeding is a parent's responsibility and only they should decide.[26] Others hold that babies fading away dehydrated and starving is morally repugnant and even against the Hippocratic principle since it produces more harm than good.[27]

I would now like to ask: why wasn't Baby 1 actively euthanized? The obvious answer is that it is *illegal* in the jurisdiction where the story happened. This was the state where Dr. Kevorkian was arrested for helping patients to die. After a *referendum*, assisted suicide and active euthanasia were rejected. That option was then not open to the medical team. But the relevant *ethical* question is this: is active non-voluntary euthanasia always immoral? Some bioethicists believe this would be the best option in these types of cases.[28] Apparently, undertaking only "palliative" care, that is, continuing fluids but no nutrition, just prolongs the dying process and makes Baby 1's suffering an unnecessary way of taking life. Certainly, the parents and the community were also in distress passively waiting for her to die. Actually, the chosen course of action seems to produce more harm than good.

To reach a reasonable conclusion on this issue, it is perhaps necessary to examine further the moral and epistemic status of "*primum*" in the non-maleficence principle. As we saw in the previous chapter, there is a huge discussion about which principle comes first: non-maleficence or beneficence

---

[26] In the famous case of Terri Schiavo, Pope John Paul II stated: "I should like particularly to underline how the administration of water and food, even when provided by artificial means, always represents a *natural means* of preserving life, not a *medical act*. Its use, furthermore, should be considered, in principle, *ordinary* and proportionate, and as such morally obligatory, insofar as and until it is seen to have attained its proper finality, which in the present case consists in providing nourishment to the patient and alleviation of his suffering." In: Arthur Caplan, James McCartney and Dominic Sisti, *The Case of Terri Schiavo*, (New York: Prometheus Books, 2006), 133. Thus, if Baby 1 had been in a Catholic hospital, she would probably not have had her nutrition withdrawn.

[27] James Rachels "Active and Passive Euthanasia". In: Robert Baird and Stuart Rosembaum, *Euthanasia*, (Buffalo: Prometheus Books, 1989), 45f.

[28] Helga Kuhse has, for one, argued that euthanasia is a better way to respect the interests of infants than to withdraw nutritional support. See: Helga Kuhse "Death by non-feeding: not in the baby's best interests," *F Med Humanit Bioeth* (1986), 7(2): 79-90. See also Helga Kuhse "A Modern Myth: That Letting Die is Not the Intentional Causation of Death." In: Helga Kuhse and Peter Singer, *Bioethics*, (Oxford: Blackwell, 2006), 315-328.

or autonomy. Even if we accept the reduction of the four principles we made in the last section, we still have the problem: what comes first *caring* or *respecting*? What becomes clear, however, is that both require non-maleficence, that is, doing no harm. Consequently, non-maleficence is an internal link between care & respect. That is why it is worth exploring further. How best then to apply both care & respect in the case of Baby 1? To answer this question, let me discuss the status of non-maleficence. We must bear in mind here that the paediatrician responsible for the Baby 1 case said he would commit civil disobedience instead of increasing care. He justified his decision by saying that it was against the Hippocratic Oath, but is it not against the same tradition to withdraw food and hydration? It seems clear that avoiding harm is, in some sense, the first requirement of true care: to care for someone is to prevent harm from occurring; it is to remove harm; to benefit without producing more harm etc. That is to say, no person *knows-how* to care *respectfully* if she produces more harm than good.

The Hippocratic tradition, which was the main inspiration for medical ethics for thousands of years in Western societies, clearly states, among other things, that the most basic rule for a physician or perhaps for any health professional is *at least* do no harm. This is the original formulation: "The physician must be able to tell the antecedents, know the present, and foretell the future –must mediate these things, and have two special objects in view with regard to diseases, mainly, to do good or at least [above all] to do no harm." Many think that this tradition is in opposition to a modern conception of morality based on rights, which is expressed in the principle of individual autonomy. But this is not *necessarily* so. When bioethics came into existence in the US, one interpretation of what was happening is that physicians/scientists were *disrespecting* this basic principle (first, do no harm) as the Tuskegee case clearly showed. Or, if we take a more holistic perspective, as Potter would remind us to do, humans were harming life as a whole by destroying the environment and other forms of life.

Modernity itself, despite emphasizing the importance of individual rights and justice, did not go in the opposite direction. For example, in his book *On Liberty*, John Stuart Mill, who is normally seen as a champion of individual rights, states a simple principle to show when society or government is entitled to interfere in an individual's life using physical force in the form of legal penalties or moral coercion of public opinion. The principle asserts that:

> the sole end for which mankind are warranted, individually or collectively, in interfering with the liberty of action of any of their number, is self-

> protection. That the only purpose for which power can be rightfully exercised over any member of a civilised community, against his will, is to prevent harm to others. His own good, either physical or moral, is not a sufficient warrant. He cannot rightfully be compelled to do or forbear because it will be better for him to do so, because it will make him happier, because, in the opinions of others, to do so would be wise, or even right.[29]

What seems clear from Mill's normative ethics, which most of the time is related to a morality based on individualistic rights, is that there are indeed negative rights, let us say, a right to be left alone, but society is justified in interfering in order to prevent harms to others. That is to say, caring & respecting must complement each other and non-maleficence is a clear link between them.

Preventing harm is also one of the cornerstones of law, both civil and criminal, and consequently, it is a pillar of public policy for any government. It is worth pointing out that ancient Roman Law was driven by these fundamental Ulpian rules, which can be considered legal middle level principles of a common morality: "*Iuris praecepta sunt haec: honeste vivere, alterum non laedere, sum cuique tribuere*," that is, the precepts of justice are: to live honorably, to harm no one, to give each his own. To harm no one is, then, a fundamental principle of the law and a common sense moral norm. Consequently, not doing harm is a necessary (and perhaps sufficient) condition for accountability and one of the most fundamental norms of a common morality, which must be internalized into a respectful attitude.

To clarify further the moral status of the non-maleficence norm, I would now like to mention briefly Albert Jonsen's paper "Do no Harm: Axiom of Medical Ethics" and sort out the main meanings of the Hippocratic principle. Jonsen identifies four types of usage to which the Hippocratic maxim can be put:

(i) a moral enterprise, an attempt to alleviate the distress and debilities in the lives of fellow humans out of concern for the good of those humans;
(ii) a commitment to giving due care as the maintenance and improvement of medical knowledge and skills in diagnosis and treatment;

---

[29] John Stuart Mill, *On Liberty and Other Writings*, (Cambridge: Cambridge University Press, 1994), 13. For a discussion on the relationship between utilitarianism and freedom in the book *On liberty*, see: Roger Crisp, *Mill On Utilitarianism*, (London/New York: Routledge, 1997), 173-200.

(iii) a judicious appeal to risk-benefit ratios in choices by physicians of those procedures with the best chance of success and the lowest risk of harm;

(iv) the development of a benefit-detriment equation, where 'do no harm' comes to mean inflict no harm not associated with a compensating benefit.[30]

Based on Jonsen's analysis, let me discriminate a *logical* sense of "primum" and an *ontological* one. To illustrate, a health professional is today justified in doing nothing to save an extremely premature baby with a very low APGAR score. For example: it was at the very beginning a justified omission not to save Baby 2, who was initially believed to be 22 weeks' gestation only. Thus, '*primum*' in this case can only mean that, in the *ontological sense*, a professional is justified in not starting an action which will produce only harm or do more harm than good. But if this were always the case, then there would be no way of justifying the ends of medicine since it exists to provide a service even if a little harm (e.g., Baby 2's surgery after she had been saved) is a necessary means to a greater good, that is, to cure a sick patient. Thus, in other cases, she can and must be driven by the principle of beneficence, by caring for a vulnerable patient in the sense analyzed in the previous section. Thus, "*primum non nocere*" cannot have an absolute status in the *logical* sense.

Albert Jonsen uses his analysis of the axiom of medical ethics, specially (ii), that is, the *due care* standard, to hold what he calls "a paradoxical use" of the general principle, namely "I would suggest that it is legitimate to invoke the 'do no harm' as a justification for termination of life."[31] This is important in shedding some light on what to do in the case of Baby 1. This view is shared by other important bioethicists, for instance, by Tristram Engelhardt.[32] He wrote: "The concept of injury for continuance of existence, the proposed analogue of the concept of the tort for wrongful life presupposes that life can be of a negative value such that

---

[30] Albert Jonsen, "Do No Harm: Axiom of Medical Ethics." In Stuart F. Spicker and Tristram Engelhardt, *Philosophical and Medical Ethics*, (Dordrecht: Reidel, 1977), 29f.

[31] Albert Jonsen, "Do No Harm: Axiom of Medical Ethics," in Stuart F Spicker and Tristram Engelhardt, *Philosophical and Medical Ethics*, (Dordrecht: Reidel, 1977), 39.

[32] Tristram Engelhardt "Ethical Issues in Aiding the Death of Young Children" in Robert Baird and Stuart Rosembaum, *Euthanasia*, (Buffalo: Prometheus Books, 1989), 148. See also his book *The Foundations of Bioethics* (Oxford: Oxford University Press, 1996), 270-1, for a similar view.

the medical maxim *primum non nocere* ("first do no harm") would require not sustaining life." Thus, the Hippocratic principle can be invoked to take a life. This is also the sense of compassionate death. The fundamental ethical question is *how* best to do that, that is, by killing or letting die?

Having clarified the status of "do no harm," it is necessary also to point out that there are many kinds of harm: physical injury (pain, disability, death, etc.), emotional abuse (humiliation, coercion, etc.), spiritual offense (mental suffering), etc. There is, of course, *moral* harm when care and respect are not provided. I do not need to make a complete typology here to recognize that all kinds of harm are bad in themselves. What counts as physical harm may be an objective fact, but it is unclear whether some kinds of harm do not depend on a personal assessment. Which is worse, physical or spiritual harm? The answer depends on a person's values related to particular moral systems. For this reason, there seems to be no *a priori* criterion to rank kinds of harm. That is why *a* common, sharable morality, based on respectful care must take into consideration most of the time what the patient herself considers to be harmful in her life. Moreover, even if there is an objective way of establishing that health is a good for anyone belonging to any particular moral system, there is a further question of the place it occupies in a person's axiological system in relation to other goods. As we have seen, reasons to care are also, in some sense, agent-relative. To illustrate with the Baby 1 case: which course of action, namely *keeping her alive, killing her* or *letting her die* produces more harm than good?

The problem of putting the patient's welfare over autonomy, as Laine Ross pointed out, "is that it assumes that what is in the patient's welfare is an objective fact that can be deduced by the physician."[33] As we have seen, that opens the door for paternalistic actions. But, in the past years, it has become clear that one has to balance the patient's welfare, especially his health, with other values. Consider Ross' illustration, "A Jehovah's Witness patient refuses blood transfusion not because the transfusion is not medically in her best interest, but because salvation is in her best interest, all things considered, and she is willing to compromise her medical best interest for her overall best interest."[34] Let me ask: is it irrational to refuse treatment? Or, on the contrary: is it irrational to want more care even in adverse circumstances such as the Baby 1 case we are discussing? There

---

[33] Laine Ross, "What is Wrong with the Physician Charter of Professionalism" (*The Hastings Center Report*. V. 36, n.4., 2006), 19.

[34] Laine Ross "What is Wrong with the Physician Charter of Professionalism" (*The Hastings Center Report*. V. 36, n.4., 2006), 19.

seems to be no ultimate, absolutely right answer to these questions. Both killing and letting die seem to be expressions of compassionate care.

To finish this chapter, let us then return to the idea of *a* common, sharable morality. At this point, it seems that there is no *ultimate* answer we can provide for the best course of action in Baby 1's case. First, she could perhaps be saved by an intestine transplantation or, perhaps, by stem cell therapy etc. This would certainly be experimental. Now, since she did not have a real second opinion, we will perhaps never know. Second, regarding the best way of taking life, Baby 1's death could occur by actively intervening and killing the patient or by "passively" waiting for her to die. In the first case, a physician could cause life to end through a special act, say by giving an injection of potassium chloride. In the second case, by discontinuing therapy, a health professional permits death to occur by omitting an act, for example, by not feeding or not resuscitating. The question is whether this particular omission is justified or not.

Now, since there is no theoretical consensus whether artificial nutrition is a parent's or a doctor's prerogative and whether killing and letting die are significantly different, we may have no way of settling this issue once and for all. Thus, apparently, *a* common, *sharable* morality, must make room for different decisions. That is to say, for parents willing to see their premature babies pass away quickly, medicine must provide better options than the one currently practiced, including in the Baby 1 case. In this sense, it is not true, *pace* Gert, Cluver, Clouser and many other bioethicists, that *a* common morality must forbid killing. If this is the case, we must also reject the idea that euthanasia cannot be legalized. Consider Beauchamp and Childress' reasons for forbidding it:

> … the belief that euthanasia is morally justified for terminally ill infants who face uncontrollable pain and suffering is consistent with the belief that the government should legally prohibit such euthanasia on grounds that it would not possible to control abuses if it were legalized.[35]

But how can euthanasia be morally justified and yet legally prohibited? To avoid abuses? I believe that the very opposite is the case: abuses occur because it is practised despite being illegal.

Beauchamp and Childress may, however, be right in claiming that the distinction between killing and letting die is flawed.[36] According to them,

---

[35] Tom L. Beauchamp and James F. Childress, *Principles of Biomedical Ethics*, (New York/Oxford: Oxford University Press, 2013), 10.

[36] Tom L. Beauchamp and James F. Childress, *Principles of Biomedical Ethics*, (New York/Oxford: Oxford University Press, 2013), 177.

despite the fact that in medicine, in law, in ethics, etc. a highly influential view is that a physician intentionally forgoing a medical technology is letting die if and only if an underlying disease or injury causes death, it is the patient's authorization that makes taking life acceptable or not. Thus, it is the authorization that determines the morality of the action. Withdrawing treatment from a patient is not, therefore, morally justifiable unless the patient has made an informed decision authorizing the withdrawal. If this is the case then both killing and letting die may be morally acceptable. In other words, a *common* morality must discriminate what is good (e.g., caring) and right (e.g., respect) for everyone and what can be *sharable* by accepting differences according to divergent moral systems (e.g., either killing or letting die).

I will return to this argument after presenting practical cognitivism as a meta-ethical substitute for the intuitionists' assumptions in the predominant theory and as the basis for a respectful caring attitude. I hope to offer an alternative for grounding *a* common, *sharable* morality on the idea that we must *know-how* to care *respectfully*. This will be presented in the next chapter. Afterwards, I will return to the Baby 1 story to say what respectful care would require in clearer terms.

CHAPTER FIVE

KNOWING HOW TO CARE RESPECTFULLY

We humans are, as social beings, care-dependent creatures and this is true of other non-human animals as well. From the very moment we are born (or even before), we need all sorts of care to meet our basic needs: we must be fed, clothed, sheltered and protected from many kinds of harm. Baby 1 and Baby 2 are examples of our extreme vulnerability and interdependence. As infants, we need to learn how to become ordinary humans by walking, talking, playing, socializing etc. all activities mastered –or not– by training/practicing and other forms of educational care. Even as adults, as autonomous agents, we not only care for others, but we need constantly to look after ourselves, so self-care plays a vital role. Later in life most of us will probably become very vulnerable, and will need to be cared for again.

Caring may, however, go wrong in many ways. For one thing, the care may be insufficient to meet the basic needs of the cared-for. It may even be a cause of negligence or malpractice. Moreover, it may degenerate into forms of paternalism when the one-caring imposes her own views of the good on a vulnerable individual, for instance, a parent on a teenager learning how be independent; a scientist on a research subject; a doctor or a nurse on a patient in need of medical attention and so forth. Besides, caring may generate anxiety, that is, be accompanied by negative feelings that compromise the wellbeing of the one-caring. An important question then arises: under which conditions can we say that the one-caring *knows-how to care* in a proper way, for instance, respectfully?

In this chapter, I would like to advance a meta-ethical theory, particularly to outline the main tenets of a new moral epistemology, which I call "practical cognitivism," and to explore some of its normative and practical, especially bioethical, implications. It is meant to be a substitute for the problematic intuitionist meta-ethical basis of the predominant bioethical theory, principlism. Thus, in the first part, I will argue for the thesis that there is moral knowledge (*pace* ethical skepticism and non-cognitivism) and that it is best understood in terms of knowing-how. That is to say, moral knowledge cannot be analyzed purely in the traditional terms of knowing-that, namely as justified belief in a true proposition. The fundamental idea is that one knows-how to act morally or knows-how to be a certain kind of person etc. only if she is *capable of* following the right normative standards (hereafter, simply norms). In the second part, I will look for ways of integrating two expressions of moral knowing-how, namely caring & respecting into a coherent normative theory making sense of our moral life. I will show that *respectful care* must be a central ingredient of such a normative theory. I will then, in the next chapter, illustrate how respectful care may transform some of our current bioethical practices.

5.1 The need for a new moral epistemology

From the very first chapter onwards, we have seen the need for a new moral epistemology for bioethics. For instance, in neonatology, doctors did not *know-how* to apply the Baby Doe guidelines. The discussions on the philosophical foundations of bioethics in the previous chapters (principlism, autonomism, beneficence-in-trust, common morality theories etc.) showed that something is missing. It is time then to try to build up better foundations for bioethics. Even nowadays, we are still in a state of moral uncertainty. We need a new moral epistemology to guide us. In this section, I will present the main tenets of *practical cognitivism* as a substitute for the intuitionist foundations of the predominant theory in bioethics, which, as we have seen, generates tensions and dilemmas.

To start with, consider another real life bioethical case:

> Baby 3 was born on March 1, 2009 at the midwife-led maternity unit Y, in the UK, after 41 weeks of "low risk" pregnancy. Thus, Baby 3 was *not* a premature baby. Two weeks before, however, the mother had complained that her baby was not moving as much. She also said that she was feeling unwell. She was examined, but nothing was identified. At this point, it would have been normal for care professionals to discuss whether she should continue with the plan to give birth at a midwife-led unit. There is no evidence, however, that any risk assessment took place. When the baby was born, she was cold and floppy and needed medical attention, yet the midwife placed her into a cold cot. Baby 3 was in a hypothermic state with signs of respiratory distress. It was only after two hours that an ambulance was called. She was transferred to a hospital to be reviewed by a paediatrician. The ambulance service refused to treat Baby 3's mother as a priority, and told her she may have to wait for transport to be with her dying daughter. It was later revealed that Baby 3 had been suffering from anaemia caused by a substantial foetal-maternal haemorrhage. Baby 3 died later that day in the hospital. She would have had a chance of surviving

had she been delivered in a hospital where she could have had a blood transfusion or any other experimental procedure or treatment.

These are the basic *facts* of the case. Some *ethical* questions are: did Baby 3 receive the care she was entitled to? If not, is this not disrespectful to *her* as a human being? How may one deliver the proper care Baby 3 was entitled to? Did Baby 3 wrongly die an avoidable death?

One of the main problems underlying insufficient, negligent care, or even supercare, that is, a paternalistic form of "caring" is, most likely, a misunderstanding regarding the very kind of knowledge that is required to look after a vulnerable being properly. An incompetent carer, we might say, must *know* better. I believe this is the case not only in the technical sense, for instance, knowing-how to make a reliable diagnosis, but also in the moral sense. In this section, then, I will argue that caring presupposes a practical kind of knowledge, namely knowing-how and not only knowing-that. The classical intuitionist meta-ethics of the predominant theory presupposes that moral knowledge is a form of knowing-that, that is, of having justified beliefs in true propositions. Now, even in philosophy, knowledge is sometimes defined in reductivistic ways obfuscating the nature of practical ways of understanding and acting. As Gilbert Ryle pointed out,[1] this is a prejudice of the "intellectualist doctrine," which tries to define intelligence in terms of apprehension of truths instead of apprehension of truth in terms of intelligence. We need, in order to avoid this inversion, to sort out a new kind of moral epistemology.

Practical cognitivism is the epistemic thesis that there is moral knowledge and that it is best understood in terms of knowing-how and not only in terms of knowing-that. The main idea is that a sound moral epistemology reveals that moral knowledge is mainly a matter of knowing-how to follow appropriate normative standards. Thus, a practical cognitivist does not deny that there is also moral knowing-that, for instance, that one must care for her daughter's wellbeing or that causing more harm than good is wrong (there are, as we will see soon, many moral

---

[1] Gilbert Ryle, *The Concept of Mind*, (New York/London: Routledge, 2009), 16. As I argued elsewhere (2008a), both Kant and Wittgenstein faced the problem that the application of a rule, for instance a moral one such as "Do not incapacitate patients", may be possible only if it is guided by another rule "Do no harm", which should, in turn, be guided by a new rule (e.g., do no more harms than benefits) and so on *ad infinitum*. To avoid this problem, both philosophers held that we need *training* through *examples* in order to develop *practical judgment*. That is why knowing-how becomes fundamental. It does not follow that we must be sceptical about the role of principles in justifying rules.

language-games), but rather argues that something else is needed: one must also *know-how* to do that. That is to say, practical cognitivism points out that there is more than one kind of knowledge and does not try to *reduce* moral knowing-how to knowing-that. Moral knowledge needs also to be clearly distinguished from other kinds of knowing-how, for instance, artisan skills, mere prudence etc. Thus, let me sort out the main features of this new moral epistemology. Hopefully, it will help us to understand what went wrong in the case of Baby 3 (and in the previously discussed cases) and to avoid similar cases happening again. I will examine this bioethical case in a more detailed way later, after establishing the basic ingredients of practical cognitivism.

To start with, let me sort out a provisory analysis of knowing-how. In order to do so, I will use Wittgenstein's project of a philosophical grammar, that is, his remarks on the rules for using the word 'know' as being closely related to that of 'can' and 'be able to' and, especially, his rule-following considerations.[2] I will explore some implications of his rule-following remarks for ethics, but I will not commit myself to the view that the moral life exclusively comprises rules. A moral system may indeed also include sentiments, rights, emotions, obligations, traits of character, values etc., as we will see regarding respectful care. Not all these elements need to be explained by referring to rules or be reduced to them. But moral rules do play a fundamental role in *guiding* a person's behaviour, in discriminating *right from wrong*, in *justifying* or in giving reasons for actions and so on. Consequently, they are a necessary condition for holding persons accountable.

What is knowledge after all? Is knowledge always related to a propositional attitude, that is, having a justified belief? This seems not to be the case. In Wittgenstein's own words: "But there is also *this* use of the word "to know": we say "Now I know!" –and similarly "Now I can do it!" and "Now I understand!"[3] Thus, to have knowledge is not simply a matter of having justified, true beliefs, but, more importantly, in the practical sense, of being capable of effectively doing something, for instance,

[2] Ludwig Wittgenstein, *Philosophical Investigations*, (Oxford: Blackwell, 1999), §185-243. For a comprehensive commentary on the *Philosophical Investigations*, especially on rule-following considerations see: Gordon Baker and Peter Hacker, *Wittgenstein Rules, Grammar and Necessity*, (Oxford: Wiley Blackwell, 2014). It shows why a communitarian and particularist reading of Wittgenstein is wrong refuting, for instance, the casuistic approach to bioethical problems presented in the first chapters of this work.

[3] Ludwig Wittgenstein, *Philosophical Investigations*, (Oxford: Blackwell, 1999), §151.

mastering a technique such as handwriting, playing chess, performing a piano piece and so on. All these activities are rule-governed practices we learn to do well by training/practicing.

Despite the fact that providing a comprehensive taxonomy of all sorts of knowledge is beyond the limits of this work, I would like now to make some further distinctions, especially between *tacit* and *explicit* knowing-how. On the one hand, a person has implicit, non-codified, knowing-how when she performs an activity without having reflected on the norms involved. On the other hand, explicit knowing-how requires mastering the principles and rules constitutive of such an activity. Now, procedural knowledge, most skills, moral knowledge etc. are subtypes of *explicit* knowing-how. Procedural knowledge or knowing-how to perform a task well, which is also sometimes referred to as "imperative knowledge," involves mastering explicit norms, for instance, a child learning how to count using her fingers. Moreover, skills are also an expression of a special kind of knowledge, which is not only propositional. If we understand a skill as a learned ability with pre-defined goals, then it is best defined as a subspecies of knowing-how. There are, of course, all sorts of skills: psychological, social etc. To illustrate: professional interaction with patients requires learning effective rules for communication. It is crucial, however, to distinguish skills from moral knowledge as the latter manifests itself in virtues. In an Aristotelian vein, we may say that virtues are not just skills, which are quick in operation but require deliberation and choice. Unfortunately, I cannot pursue further this issue here.[4] Other differences between moral knowledge and the other kinds of knowing-how will become apparent in the next section.

Professional knowledge may involve all sorts of knowledge. The exercise of modern medicine, for instance, requires different kinds of expertise. It certainly needs factual knowledge, especially scientific knowledge such as provided by chemistry, biology etc., for example, knowing that the blood is pumped by the heart to the arteries, the arterioles and the capillaries, and returns in the venous system to be oxygenated in the lungs. However, since health care professions also have a practical component, their goal is doing and not just knowing. Doing something involves knowing-how, for instance, to bypass coronary arteries, which is a technical kind of knowledge. They need practical skills too, which may improve upon new procedures for bypassing arteries. Moral knowledge is also required since what *can* be done, perhaps *must not* be done. More

[4] For an excellent collection of essays on kinds of knowing-how see: John Bengson and Marc Moffett, *Knowing How*, (Oxford: Oxford University Press, 2011).

importantly, one needs to *know how* to follow normative standards. Medicine can even be considered a form of wisdom, that is, it requires practical rationality and not only scientific knowledge. This is why, as was recently pointed out by Julian Savulescu, philosophy is really important for bioethics.[5]

I would now like to present a definition of explicit knowing-how.[6] It can be done in these terms: it is an acquired capacity to follow normative standards. This definition establishes a rule for using the expression "she knows-how" distinguishing its right from wrong uses. The above definition contains elements which clearly show that knowing-how is irreducible to knowing-that. I believe that people like Jason Stanley are mistaken in claiming the reducibility of knowing-how to knowing-that. Recently, he has argued, even against the strong evidence from neuroscience, that procedural knowledge is a kind of knowing-that.[7] This is not the case since procedural knowledge, that is, knowing-how to perform a task well, involves above all the mastering of norms. One may know-that she must care for her daddy, but do not know-how to look after him respectfully. That is to say: *knowing-that is not sufficient to knowing-how*. To recognize this point, imagine you are going to learn a new game. You need certainly to practice *how* to follow the constitutive rules and not just learn *that* they are A, B, C... Thus, knowing-how is not just a matter of having beliefs in true propositions; it is a matter of mastering the norms necessary to perform activities, that is, being able to apply them effectively to get the desired results. It does not follow, then, that there is no need for knowing-that or that one is, *pace* Ryle, more fundamental than the other. On the contrary, knowing-how may involve knowing-that. The basic point is just that they represent two different kinds of knowledge, which may well be characterized in terms of the distinction between practical and theoretical philosophy: the former deals with what *ought to be*; the latter is an inquiry into what *is* the case. And this is arguably the most important advantage of explaining moral knowledge in terms of knowing-how, namely "the problem of normativity" (the way "*ought-ness*" is *sui generis* and yet compatible with the natural world) is solved by

---

[5] Julian Savulescu, "Bioethics: Why Philosophy is Essential for Progress." *Journal of Medical Ethics*, 2015, (41): 28.

[6] I offer a conceptual analysis of knowing-how, in analogy with knowing-that, in my paper "Practical Cognitivism" (2008b, 7(2)), 323-339). Both kinds of knowledge, however, differ from knowledge by acquaintance (e.g., in sentences such as "I know Steve.").

[7] Jason Stanley, *Know How*, (Oxford: Oxford University Press, 2011), 150f. I will not discuss here counter-examples to the definition of knowing-that.

introducing it right inside our analytical model. That is to say, it shows that norms are irreducible to facts.

If this is the case, then there is an important implication for current meta-ethical debates: we must, so to speak, turn the tables. Most present day discussions are contaminated by the single (and false) presupposition that either there is moral knowledge or there is not; however, both sides, most cognitivists and non-cognitivists alike, think exclusively in terms of knowing-that. For instance, an intuitionist such as G. E. Moore (and many present day intuitionists) has many problems in showing us how such knowledge is possible, so he finds himself postulating strange faculties or subscribing to queer entities.[8] Many cognitivists follow the same path by trying to reduce ethics to empirical investigations naturalizing morality and thus committing the naturalistic fallacy. But, on the other hand, non-cognitivists do not come out with better solutions despite the fact that they are successful in showing us that not all moral judgments are propositions in the strictest sense.[9] The shared mistake is to assume just one kind of knowledge either in affirming (cognitivists) or denying it (non-cognitivists). Therefore, what we need is to twist the debate in the direction of knowing-how.

I will now go back to practical cognitivism and deal with more epistemic issues surrounding it. First, there is the question of objectivity. Since norms are the basic ingredient of *explicit* knowing-how (as propositions are for knowing-that), it seems clear that the discussion of whether moral judgments are objective or not, according to a practical cognitivist, must be related to the kind of entity *norms* (principles, rules etc.) are. In this sense, it is not difficult to recognize that norms are objective in their own way; that is, if they are clearly formulated, they co-ordinate the behaviour of all agents. To say "all persons must not cause more harms than benefits" does not express subjective feelings, but objectively prescribes a specific kind of action. That is why a non-cognitivist is wrong: following a rule (*not merely acting in accordance with it*) is a cognitive state. A norm presents a standard for agents to act accordingly. Thus, objectivity in ethics has nothing to do with finding queer objects "out there," which supposedly must correspond to moral

---

[8] For a critical comment on this point, see my dissertation "Intrinsic Value: Analysing Moore's Ethics" (University of Bristol, 2000).

[9] Wittgenstein himself, in the *Tractatus*, declared "there are no propositions in ethics" (6.42). For a discussion of Wittgenstein's ethics in the *Tractatus* see my paper "What We Cannot Say, we Can and Must Speak About," in Marek, J. C. and Reicher M. (eds.), *Experience and Analysis*, (Kichberg am Wechsel: WAB archives, XII), 89-91.

terms or concepts. On the contrary, it is a matter of recognizing that moral norms direct behaviour. Thus, moral norms such as the fundamental principles of bioethics (e.g., *first, do no harm*), which are constitutive ingredients of caring & respecting, are objective in this sense and once they are internalized they convert into attitudes, for instance, a respectful caring one, which are not subjective either.

The question relating to the philosophical problem of truth may have a similar (dis)solution. What we must mainly be concerned with, from a cognitivist point of view, is not whether all our moral judgments *correspond* to facts in the world, but whether a system of norms is *coherent* and helps us achieve our goals. That is to say, we may assume here a redundancy approach to truth. As Wittgenstein noted while commenting on Broad's three-fold classification of theories of truth as correspondence, coherence and pragmatic: "We can say that the word ['truth'] has at least three different meanings; but it is mistaken to assume that any one of these theories can give the whole grammar of how we use the word, or endeavour to fit into a single theory cases which do not seem to agree with it."[10] I believe that contemporary philosophy has overlooked the importance of this remark. The truth of moral sentences depends on the language-game in which they occur.

To recognize this point, let me examine more deeply Wittgenstein's notion of language-games applying it to moral language. A moral system may include the following language-games:

(i) *imperative* moral language-games (comprising sentences enunciating principles –general guides for action– such as "do no harm" and particular rules which prescribe or make permissible specific acts, for instance, "do not cause physical injury," "do not cause offence" etc.); these normative games are linked to our practices of coordinating human relationships and some are the bases for legal institutions; particular rules may be said to be *true* if we accept principles and they cohere with them;

(ii) *evaluative* moral language-games (sentences to assess certain forms of behaviour, attitudes or qualities of an agent's character such as "Peter is a good fellow"); these evaluative language-games are linked to our practices of judging what we do and what kind of person we are and help us to establish ends for our institutions and lives; these sentences may be *true* in the correspondent sense if

[10] *Apud* Ray Monk, *Ludwig Wittgenstein*, (London, Vintage, 1991), 322.

they describe accurately what a person is, for instance, whether an agent *is* an honest person;

(iii) *performative* moral language-games (sentences which themselves express actions we do, for instance, a person at her wedding saying "I promise to ...."); such judgements are linked to our practices of creating culture; these sentences can be said to be *true* in a pragmatic sense.

There might be several other kinds of moral language-games. We may say that there are *deliberative* moral language-games (when we are figuring out the best course of action or the best results); *laudatory* moral language-games (when we encourage people to act in certain ways...); *imputative* moral language-games (when we ascribe certain actions to an agent, holding her accountable). There is no need to try to present a complete list here.[11] The main theoretical advantage of applying the concept of language-games in ethics is to get us to realize that particular words do not have a moral meaning in themselves, but they may *function* as such, for instance, the word "no" can be used in a normative-language-game as a moral imperative. That is to say, the atomistic investigation of the meanings of 'good', 'right' etc. considered in isolation is misleading and we are better off with a systemic approach to moral language using the notion of language-games.

Let me now make clearer why the acceptance of this multiplicity of *moral* language-games does not imply radical relativism. First, I was using different meanings of 'true', relating it to different kinds of language-games. Thus, it is important to stress that Wittgenstein rejects a *theory* of truth, but not that moral judgements are true or false. Thus, if we accept the *prima facie* principle of non-maleficence "do no harm" as true, then we must also follow particular rules such as "do not cause pain," "do not cause suffering" and so on. In this sense, norms form a coherent web of guiding directives for our actions. In a minimalist sense, they can be said to be true, just as it may well be true that an evaluative moral judgement is in accordance with what is stated.

Norms are, then, objective and may even be said to be true, but that is not to argue that norms are not revisable. A practical cognitivist may well be a fallibilist and not a foundationist about the justification of accepting

---

[11] For further discussion of Wittgenstein's developments in ethics see my "Practical Cognitivism: Knowing-how to Follow a Rule" in Christian Kanzian *et al.* (eds.), *Realism, Relativism and Constructivism*, (Kichberg am Wechsel: WAB archives, v. XXIII), 53-55. For a discussion whether to accept that the multiplicity of moral languages implies relativism, see my reply (2013a) to Sanfèlix Vidarte.

norms. That is to say, as for beliefs, we may constantly revise our norms, correcting them, perfecting them. For instance, the principle of non-maleficence can be rewritten in terms of "do no more harm than benefit", asking a subject of scientific research or a patient herself to say what counts as harm. The rules related to it may also be rewritten and improved. This adjustment is an ongoing project. Does that imply radical relativism? I will try to show now that this is not the case.

All mentioned moral language-games, and possibly many others, are descriptions of how Wittgenstein characterizes our lifeform (*Lebensform*), that is, how we, as humans, use moral language. In this sense, they are part of a *common* morality. Without engaging in a scholastic debate about whether the singular or the plural sense of '*Lebensform*(*en*)' is more relevant, I will try to show that despite the fact that Wittgenstein uses both, he is more concerned with our *human* lifeform, analysing it in comparison to other forms such as the leonine, the canine, the imagined spherical Martians, or even imagined tribes with non-human-feelings and alien concepts etc. for philosophical purposes. That is to say, he wants, for instance, to spell out conditions of sense (e.g., regularity in using terms, propositions etc.) expunging metaphysical statements. Here is the main evidence: "What is true or false is what human beings *say*; and it is in their *language* that human beings agree. This is agreement not in opinions, but rather in lifeform."[12] This provides a more basic kind of agreement, not merely a Rawlsian kind of consensus. Here is another: "Shared human behaviour (*die gemeinsamemenschliche Handlungsweise*) is the system of reference by means of which we interpret an unknown language."[13] Thus, I believe that the expression *Lebensform* refers mainly to the human lifeform, especially to what is common to all of us, for instance, we are care-dependent creatures. Caring is as much a part of our natural history as playing, talking etc. Therefore, Wittgenstein does not subscribe to extreme forms of ethical relativism. On the contrary, he shows us a way of overcoming it. If this is true, then we must also reject the particularist interpretation of his (bio)ethics presented in the second chapter (e.g., Toulmin's casuistry) and other relativistic readings.

In order to recognize this point, I would like to recall the distinction made by Robert Arrington between *empirical*-moral-propositions and

---

[12] Ludwig Wittgenstein, *Philosophical Investigations*, (Oxford: Blackwell, 1999), § 241.

[13] Ludwig Wittgenstein, *Philosophical Investigations*, (Oxford: Blackwell, 1999), § 206.

grammatical-moral-propositions.[14] If one says "It is wrong for Jack and Jill to have pre-marital sex," this proposition might be true or false depending on particular circumstances. Here we find a place for a Wittgensteinian kind of limited pluralism allowing diversity, for instance, in sexual matters. But if one says that "Lying is wrong!" one is just sorting out the meaning of 'lying,' that is, expressing a grammatical proposition. The same is true of "Rape is wrong": it is bad in itself.

Let me now introduce, recalling Wittgenstein's famous river-bed analogy,[15] a further distinction between:

(i) *hinge*-grammatical-moral-propositions;
(ii) *non-hinge*-grammatical-moral-propositions.

The second kind of proposition establishes the meaning of particular moral concepts such as truth-telling, but the former would give us *the grammar of morality* itself. For instance, a fundamental *hinge*-grammatical-moral-proposition seems to be "good is to be done and evil avoided." From a Wittgensteinian point of view, it is simply *nonsensical* to say that a member of our lifeform behaves morally by producing more harms than benefits. The above *hinge*-grammatical-moral-proposition coheres with a set of particular true bioethical rules such as "do not cause suffering" etc. Another *hinge*-grammatical-moral-proposition seems to be "respect persons" given that a 'person' can be defined as a rule-following being. Empirical bioethical propositions such as "respect the privacy of others", "obtain consent for interventions with patients" etc. cohere with this principle. Thus, to disrespect persons seems, from a Wittgensteinian point of view, to be annihilating morality itself; it is simply *unintelligible*

---

[14] Robert Arrington, "A Wittgensteinian Approach to Ethical Intuitionism" in Stratton-Lake, P. (ed.), *Ethical Intuitionism*, (Oxford: Clarendon Press, 2002), 271f.

[15] Wittgenstein wrote: "It might be imagined that some propositions, of the form of empirical propositions, were hardened and functioned as channels for such empirical propositions as were not hardened but fluid; and that this relation altered with time, in that fluid propositions hardened, and hard ones became fluid. The mythology may change back into a state of flux; the river-bed of thoughts may shift. But I distinguish between the movement of the waters on the river-bed and the shift of the bed itself; though there is not a sharp division of the one from the other. ... And the bank of that river consists partly of hard rock, subject to no alteration or only to an imperceptible one, partly of sand, which now is one place now in another gets washed away or deposited." Ludwig Wittgenstein, *On Certainty*, (New York: Harper and Row, 1972), §96-99

for our lifeform. Therefore, care & respect are the hinges of moral life, everything else moving around them.

These two hinge-grammatical-moral-propositions may be considered the river-bed of our moral thoughts and the rules which follow from them the river-waters of our moral life. This web of norms shows that there are clear limits to what one may call "ethical" or "moral". If this is the case, then it urges us to reject most post-modern readings of Wittgenstein's moral philosophy as representing some sort of relativism. Denying a hinge-grammatical-moral-proposition makes morality unintelligible for our *human* lifeform. No reasonable person would do that. They provide the bases for *a common* morality, allowing for a variety of divergences of particular matters. Consequently, it is possible to accept these differences (e.g., on having or not pre-marital sex) in a *sharable* morality, with common hinge principles (e.g., doing no more harms than good). In meta-ethical terms: descriptive pluralism does not entail ethical relativism.

A practical cognitivist may, then, be considered a realist in the relational sense. That is to say, it is compatible with what Peter Railton calls "an objectified subjective interest" for an individual A^+. Railton describes A^+ in this way: "give to an actual individual *A* unqualified cognitive and imaginative powers, and full factual and nomological information about his physical and psychological constitution, capacities, circumstances, history, and so on."[16] I would now like to add, complementing Railton, that A^+ must also have *knowing-how* to a high, excellent degree. In other words, knowing-how presupposes the exercise of full capacities in order to act morally or have the appropriate attitudes. What counts as real (e.g., the ingredients of one's welfare), then, is what is established from the point of view of A^+ and not from an independent realm of values "out there".

If this conclusion is right, we have found the path to follow in order to construct a normative ethics based on knowing-how to care. There are certainly different kinds of knowing-how and also different kinds of care, for instance, natural care and moral care. There are, perhaps, only family resemblances between them. Thus, it is important to distinguish *moral* knowing-how (e.g., to care for someone for *her* own sake) from non-moral knowing-how (e.g., caring for a particular book). In this sense, I would like to adopt here a specific use of the word 'moral', which is after all a common sense use that is also assumed in many empirical studies of morality, namely as a synonym for altruistic behaviour. To be more

[16] Peter Railton, *Facts, Values, and Norms*, (New York: Cambridge University Press, 2003), 11.

precise, and given that there is also the morally relevant case of self-care, I would like to use the following criteria to distinguish moral from non-moral kinds of knowing-how: in the former case, it presupposes a special kind of valuation, namely the ascription of intrinsic value; in the latter, there is no such assumption. This is the domain of morality: from Aristotle's conception of *praxis*, through Kant's *definition* of a categorical imperative, to Wittgenstein's notion of *absolute values*, morality is a domain composed of intrinsic values. Self-care and caring for others are, consequently, expressions of the intrinsic valuing of a vulnerable being.

I will from now on use this criterion to distinguish moral norms from non-moral ones. For this purpose, I will refer to Wittgenstein's *Tractatus*. He wrote: "When an ethical law of the form, 'Thou shalt …', is laid down, one's first thought is, 'And what if I do not do it?' … There must be indeed some kind of ethical reward and ethical punishment, but they must reside in the action itself."[17] The distinctive feature of a moral law is, then, that it commands an action as good *in itself*. In other words, a moral rule is a categorical not a hypothetical norm. In his *Lecture of Ethics*, Wittgenstein makes the distinction between a *relative* and an *absolute* use of moral words. His example of an absolute use is this: suppose I had told somebody here a preposterous lie and he came up to me and said "You're behaving like a beast" and then I said "I know I'm behaving badly, but I don't want to behave any better", could he then say "Ah, then that's all right"? Certainly not; he would say "Well, you *ought* to want to behave better". It seems clear that moral knowledge relates to an intrinsic valuation: *the ascription of what is good in itself or right in itself*. In this sense, there is no priority between 'right' and 'good' because both may be defined in terms of value. This is important in realizing how we can overcome the dichotomy between deontology and teleology/consequentialism in normative ethics: both rightness and goodness are instantiations of intrinsic value. I will argue for this in the next section, showing how care & respect can be integrated into a single normative ethics, for instance, when one *knows-how* to care respectfully. Consequently, the moral epistemology needed for grounding respectful care is now presented under the meta-ethics of practical cognitivism, which provided also the grounds for *a* common, sharable morality.

---

[17] Ludwig Wittgenstein, *Tractatus Logico-philosophicus*, (London: Routledge, 1997), 71-2 (remark 6.422).

5.2 The concept of respectful care

I would now like to illustrate in a more detailed way how practical cognitivism, that is, the epistemic theory that says that moral knowledge is best understood in terms of knowing-how, describes two important moral attitudes, namely caring & respecting. These notions are the foundations of bioethics, the field with which I am most concerned here, and are the basic building blocks of *a common, sharable* morality. Just to be clear: I am not assuming that caring & respecting are the only intrinsic valuations, but there is no doubt that they represent the kind of knowledge a practical cognitivist holds to be central to public morality, particularly in special bioethics. In this section, then, I will look for the conditions required for knowing-how to care in a respectful manner.

To start with, let me recall some previous results of this work. The predominant bioethical approach, namely the theory called "principlism" was based on the *prima facie* norms of respect for autonomy (a person's choices must be considered), non-maleficence (harm must be avoided), beneficence (more benefits than otherwise must result from our actions) and justice (a distribution is a fair one if it gives equally to equals and differently to non-equals). This approach is, meta-ethically speaking, intuitionist (there are several principles and no way of ranking them), and this may lead to arbitrary applications or to dilemmas, as perhaps Baby 3 also shows. We need a better meta-ethics for bioethics. On the other hand, if we want to avoid both paternalism (a problem for Pellegrino's model of beneficence-in-trust, which still gives too much weight to the traditional Hippocratic principles) and individualism or indifference (e.g., Engelhardt's autonomism, which gives absolute priority to personal consent), we need to integrate both care & respect to create the main core of *a common, sharable* morality in a more balanced way. This is not the idea of *the* morality as some bioethicists hold is necessary. As we saw in the last chapter, in their book *Bioethics: a Return to Fundamentals*, Gert, Culver and Clouser present, as an alternative to the predominant bioethical theory, the common morality as a public system for all, which manifests itself in different cultures, including professions. Such morality comprises several moral rules such as "don't kill" etc., which supposedly are part of all existent moral systems. This idea was incorporated into principlism by Beauchamp and Childress. Grounding principlism in common morality seems to provide a remedy for many meta-ethical intuitionist problems, however it may bring new ones. Consider, for instance, the issues involved in the end of life processes, the problems surrounding the euthanasia debate: either in prolonging life or shortening it. When the futility of any treatment is the case (a cure is not possible), a person has the moral right to refuse extraordinary means to keep her alive. In order to respect her as a person, this right must be granted, but it does not follow that she must not be cared for. How then to provide her with real respectful care? For one asking for it, *real* palliative care is the way to value her for her own sake and to show respectful care and caring respect. For those asking for assistance to die, however, the only way to value them intrinsically is to provide a dignified way of passing away, but this is something the proponents of *the* common morality argued was against the rule “don’t kill” in medical contexts. Medicine is, however, a social practice and its goals may change. Thus, it seems clear that we need to *know-how* to integrate care & respect, which comprise the four principles of the predominant normative theory in bioethics, in *a common, sharable* morality. This is the main advantage of the new moral epistemology, practical cognitivism, mainly presented in the last section.

The knowledge implicit in caring for a vulnerable individual (a human being or even a sentient non-human animal) is knowing-how to increase her wellbeing (and also prevent loss of wellbeing), not just in the technical sense of doing what must be done to cure her if she is a patient/subject of research, but also in the *moral* sense, which presupposes an intrinsic valuation: the person’s welfare must be fostered because it is good *for her* own sake. If there is no such evaluative attitude, there is no moral worth in caring for her. Here, we must also remember that there is a distinction between natural and moral care. Thus, knowing-how to act morally involves an intrinsic valuation: a person knows-how to care if she answers in the appropriate way, for instance sympathetically, to an individual’s wellbeing and acts accordingly protecting it, fostering it and so on, doing whatever is necessary *for the vulnerable’s own sake*. An ethics of care (as represented by the works of Gilligan, Noddings, Hildeman, Engster etc.) is arguably a consequence of practical cognitivism. I am not assuming here, however, the particularist assumptions generally subscribed to by most defenders of an ethics of care. In fact, a norm such as the non-maleficence principle is always applicable in any case where caring is at stake. No one *knows-how* to care if she produces more harm than benefit and, if the above criterion is the right one, no one *knows-how* to care, in the moral sense, if she does not increase an individual’s welfare or prevent loss of welfare for the *cared-for*’s *own sake*.

As we saw in the previous section, professional medical knowledge involves all sorts of expertise. Now, regarding knowing-how to care, we may also distinguish between common moral knowledge and professional moral knowledge. For this proposal, it is crucial to bear in mind the differences between *general* and *specific* care or beneficence. According to Beauchamp and Childress, specific beneficence rests on special relations, contracts, or particular commitments and it is directed at specific parties such as children, patients, etc.; on the other hand, general beneficence is directed beyond special relationships to all persons.[18] It is worth remembering that, in chapter 4, I provided an analysis of *special care* only. In this sense, health care professionals have *specific* obligations of beneficence through taking on a role. Consequently, moral knowing-how to care professionally is, in some sense, agent-relative despite the fact that, as Darwall has correctly pointed out, reasons to care are agent-neutral in the non-positional sense.

Before developing further other normative implications of practical cognitivism, let me give one more example of moral knowing-how: a person knows-how to respect another person only if she is capable of deferring to *her* rights. In other words, in order to respect another person, one needs to recognize her *as* a person (a free agent and a holder of rights and a bearer of obligations) and to revere her rights *for her* own sake. The so-called "respect for autonomy" in bioethics which amounts to self-determination may here be a particular right a person has, but there are many others. A patient, as a person, has many rights: to advocacy services, to meet with clergy, to information etc. etc. and not just to receive the necessary and basic care. It is easy to grant one right (to self-determination) forgetting other rights such as the right to be cared for, which is disrespectful; conversely, it is easy to grant the right to be cared for and to forget the right to self-determination. This is the origin of both indifference and paternalism, a problem a respectful caring attitude avoids at once. Thus, instead of respect for autonomy at the foundations of bioethics, one must think in terms of respect for persons, which is another hinge moral norm. An ethics of universal respect (as represented by the works of Tugendhat, Dworkin, Darwall etc.) may also be seen as a consequence of practical cognitivism. That is to say: a person knows-how to respect only if she recognizes the other person's rights and has the relevant moral attitude of deferring, protecting, fostering etc. them because they are *their* rights. If such intrinsic valuation is not implicit, there is no moral value in her actions even if rights are not directly violated.

If we now ask what kind of moral system we can build from practical cognitivism, one possible answer is this: on the one hand, since there is not just one single conception of wellbeing or even a single consensual set of

---

[18] Tom L. Beauchamp and James F. Childress, *Principles of Biomedical Ethics*, (New York/Oxford: Oxford University Press, 2013), 205.

claim rights, then we are bound to accept some sort of pluralism; on the other hand, if we want at the same time to avoid an extreme form of ethical relativism, then we must build up *a common, sharable* morality, which has, so to speak, a "transcendental" function: it makes possible the pacific and cooperative co-existence of persons even if they belong to different moral systems (Christians, agnostics, Buddhists, atheists and so on). Thus, *a* common, sharable morality allows for a limited kind of pluralism (e.g., to have pre-marital sex or not), although it restricts unreasonable axiological systems, for example, it does not tolerate rape. Now, respectful care & caring respect are the core of this minimalist *public* system of morality. As we have seen, both caring and respecting are expressions of intrinsically valuing an individual and/or a person and that is why they are *moral* attitudes. Despite the fact that there is no space here to argue for this in a more detailed way, I am assuming that care & respect are complementary aspects of the moral life at the foundations of what I have called "*a* common, sharable morality." In this sense, care & respect seem irreducible because they limit each other avoiding both paternalism and individualism in bioethics and in other domains of life. This remark applies to an intersubjective or social sphere, but it is also true of self-regarding concerns. That is to say, both self-respect and self-care are expressions of moral attitudes in the above defined sense.

How then can we now integrate care & respect into a solid normative ethics? Apart from principlism, there are currently important projects being carried out which are trying to overcome the dichotomy between kinds of deontology (Kantianism, contractualism) and consequentialism.[19] For instance, Derek Parfit, in *On What Matters*, proposes a Triple Theory in normative ethics holding that "an act is wrong just when such acts are disallowed by the principles that are optimific, uniquely universally willable, and not reasonably rejectable."[20] I believe that we need to amend

---

[19] Richard Hare is famous for holding a Kantian form of utilitarianism (See his paper "Could Kant Have Been a Utilitarian?" In: Richard Hare, *Sorting Out Ethics*, (Oxford: Clarendon Press, 2000), 147f.). Moreover, Jeremy Wisnewski has argued, from a Wittgensteinian point of view (as holding a *clarificatory* ethics), that we can read Kant and Mill as compatible. According to Wisnewski, a Wittgensteinian rethinking of Kant's Categorical Imperative shows that we can understand Kant as clarifying the logic of moral rationality and a Wittgensteinian rethinking of Mill's Utilitarianism shows us that Mill was mainly concerned with clarifying the constituents of human flourishing. See my review of Wisnewski's book for further comments.

[20] Derek Parfit, *On what Matters*, (Oxford: Oxford University Press, 2011), 413. In my previous works in bioethics, including the mentioned talks in Michigan on "Care & Respect", I was using a similar principle to overcome the dichotomy

Parfit's Triple Theory to include virtue ethics, as we have seen in the first chapter, the other major normative ethics in contemporary philosophy. According to virtue ethics, an agent is always obligated to, as Roger Crisp puts it, *act as the virtuous person would act.*[21] This is also a purely formal criterion as it is "optimific", "universally willable" etc. and can be incorporated into a renewed Triple Theory. Moreover, we can in this way make sense of the idea that the teleological principles at the bottom of caring (non-maleficence and beneficence) and the deontological ones at the bottom of respecting (concerning self-determination and equal share in distribution) can be united into a single "metanorm" for *a common, sharable* morality. The fundamental norm in normative ethics may then be formulated in this way:

> *First principle of normative ethics for* a *common, sharable morality:* act under norms that are optimific, uniquely universally willable and would not be rejected by a virtuous person.

Now, respectful care seems to be the kind of moral attitude that is based on norms that are optimific, universally willable and would, certainly, not be rejected by a virtuous character. Therefore, the amended Triple Theory may provide the right balance between caring & respecting, overcoming the difficulties of the predominant normative theory in bioethics and its main variations, namely autonomism and beneficence-in-trust. If this is right and we remember the state of the bioethics art reconstructed in the first chapters of this work, then we will realize that Beauchamp's utilitarian approach to bioethics, Engelhardt's deontological (contractualist) view and Pellegrino's virtue ethics model are not formally incompatible and they may, in practice, subscribe to a concept such as *respectful care.*

---

between deontological and teleological normative ethical theories and also the difficulties of principlism, namely: *Wisely apply in C_1 the principle(s) that can be generalized (applied in similar circumstances) bringing the best consequences for life and thus becoming a universal law.* Here, I chose to amend Parfit's first principle and I am more concerned with the internalization of norms (both principles and rules) into an attitude. The intuitionist problems of principlism are finally solved.

[21] Roger Crisp, *Reasons & the Good*, (Oxford: Oxford University Press, 2008), 33. For a comprehensive study of virtue ethics see: Roger Crisp and Michael Slote (eds.), *Virtue Ethics*, (Oxford: Oxford University Press, 1997).

This is perhaps the best place to point out that this first principle of ethics is based on what Roger Crisp calls "normative intuitionism".[22] This must *not* be conflated with intuitionism in Rawls' sense, which provides the meta-ethical basis for principlism in bioethics. That is to say, the first principle of the renewed Triple Theory is grasped by intuition and since such a grasp provides justification for believing it and that it cannot otherwise be reached by another methodology such as induction, then it must be assumed as self-evident. According to Crisp, normative intuition is a capacity that enables us to grasp the truth of certain *a priori* propositions as reasons for action.[23] I do agree with Roger Crisp that it is debatable whether *a priori* propositions are unconditionally necessary. Kant thought so, but contemporary developments have shown that this may not be the case. Consequently, it is perhaps better to consider them hinge-propositions in the Wittgensteinian sense spelled out above. Thus, I will here consider the first principle of ethics an *a priori* hinge-proposition capable of unifying the three main normative approaches in contemporary moral philosophy. It represents a breakthrough in normative ethics. Finally, it provides the normative foundation for respectful care in bioethics as we will see now.

I believe that we are still far from having a clear understanding of what *respectful care* actually requires in practice and perhaps the amended Triple Theory can help us to get there. This is one reason why some of our practices may go wrong and we fail to deliver proper care as the case of Baby 3 clearly shows. I hope here to make a small contribution to this topic by calling attention to some elements we need to consider in order to build this new bioethical concept, namely that of respectful care. There is little doubt that Baby 3 should not have been delivered at a midwife-led unit. This was disrespectful to the baby herself. True care needs not only good intentions or nice feelings (sympathy), but also real conditions to benefit a vulnerable individual at risk of losing her life. The attention needed to improve a patient's wellbeing, to restore her health or simply to protect her from further harm must be accompanied by effective knowledge, both scientifically and morally speaking, and by material conditions. There are many mistakes that care is subject to. Technical errors, for instance in diagnosis, are not the only ones that may occur.

[22] According to Crisp, normative intuitionism makes three main assumptions: (i) *foundationism*; (ii) *normative non-septicism* and (iii) *the autonomy of normativity*. See: Roger Crisp, *Reasons & the Good*, (Oxford: Oxford University Press, 2006), 72. As I argued previously, however, a practical cognitivist does not need to commit herself to foundationism.

[23] Roger Crisp, *Reasons & the Good*, (Oxford: Oxford University Press, 2006), 75.

There can also be moral failures. Let me then ask: under what conditions does one *know-how* to *care* for a vulnerable individual *respectfully*?

As we have seen in the first part of this chapter, knowing-how to care is not just a question of having justified, true beliefs, but requires the effective capacity of following some normative standards. Practices such as playing chess, diagnosing diseases, etc. require the development of relevant skills. In the same way, acting morally requires acquiring knowing-how, for instance, to care for a vulnerable individual *for her own sake*. Thus, caring & respecting are mastered by training/practicing in order to develop the necessary capabilities to benefit a person's wellbeing and not with informational knowledge only. Moral training consists in teaching normative standards by given examples, inculcating rules and principles, punishing wrong doings etc., so that the apprentice internalizes them up to the point that they are part of her own character. Moral education also involves learning-how to respond appropriately to the special value persons have. Only then does one know-how to act morally and will develop the relevant moral attitudes.

Moral sentiments such as sympathetic concern are also a condition of proper care. Sympathy is just a natural sharing of feelings and emotions, both negative and positive, any social animal is capable of. It is immediate and involuntary arising out of our intersubjective interactions. In the human case, it is sometimes accompanied by empathy, that is, by imaginatively placing oneself in another person's shoes and simulating how she feels. Although they are certainly essential for proper caring, sympathy and empathy may not be sufficient. Moreover, feelings are sometimes misleading and may even compromise proper care. If one allows oneself to be guided just by anxiety, one may end up acting wrongly. Thus, empathy must be tempered with reflection on what is really best to benefit the patient's wellbeing, for instance, to effectively improve her health. Recalling the case mentioned, midwives were probably very sensitive, but perhaps lacked the material conditions to effectively benefit Baby 3's wellbeing.

There is another necessary ingredient for proper care. Apart from sentiments such as sympathetic concern and empathy, the recognition of the patient as a person is essential. Without making here a detailed examination of what a person is, let us recall that a person is a rule-following being, a bearer of rights and/or obligations. Thus, a patient has not only the basic right to health assistance, but other rights as well, such as to give informed consent, to call for a second opinion, to have her privacy protected etc. As we have seen in the previous chapter, to respect a person is not only to fulfill our obligations regarding improving her health, but to be careful not to violate other rights as well. Consequently, it seems clear that in the case of Baby 3 proper care was not delivered because not all rights were respected. If the mother was complaining before giving birth, a second opinion should have been sought. In some sense, Baby 3 tragically repeats the Baby 1 story. A second opinion was not provided. Both parents and midwives should have remembered this and requested an obstetrician's review.

Another condition is necessary to give caring a full moral sense. The one-caring must benefit the cared-for because this is good for the patient's own sake. This is the right thing to do. Thus, morality requires evaluating intrinsically a vulnerable individual or a person. If the one-caring "cares" for the vulnerable out of self-interest only, then "caring" has no moral meaning. If the one-caring is only concerned with earning money or not losing her job, then caring may not only go wrong from a technical point of view, but could also represent a moral failure. Health sciences and practices, as many philosophers have argued, are moral enterprises. Therefore, to achieve its moral goal, caring needs to proceed with an intrinsic valuation.

Taking into account the results of the previous chapter (the analyses of both 'care' & 'respect') and the two sections of this one (especially, the new moral epistemology provided by practical cognitivism), we may now sum up the conditions of respectful care asserting that W *knows-how* to *care for* X *respectfully* iff:

i) W sympathizes with X, but also recognizes her as a p (person);
ii) X's wellbeing needs attention and p has, among others, a basic right to health assistance;
iii) W fulfils her obligations benefiting X for *her* own sake.

By definition, then, respectful care causes an increase in one's wellbeing or prevents a fall in welfare for one's own sake without violating other rights. It instantiates an intrinsic valuation and, consequently, it is a moral attitude. Respectful care is optimific, universally willable and would not be rejected by a virtuous person. I will apply the concept of respectful care to the Baby 3 story as well as the other cases in the next section in greater detail.

A common, sharable morality (granted, not *the* eternal and immutable morality), based on respectful care, is greatly needed nowadays for bioethics in our globalized, pluralistic society. It is also the best candidate to provide the political foundation for justifying a state and its institutional policies enforcing many forms of caring. Since discussing all these political arrangements is beyond the limits of this work, I will only refer to Engster's defence of caring as a political value. Starting with a clear list of basic needs (and basic capabilities), namely food, sanitary water, clothing, shelter, rest, a clean environment, basic medical care and protection from harms, Engster spells out reasons to institutionalize *collective* not just personal, face to face, care. According to him, some public goods such as security, clean environment etc., including medical care, can only be provided by a government-like entity.[24] He then goes on to sort out principles for a *caring* government: first and most importantly, to help individuals to meet their basic needs, including basic medical care.[25] Thus, among the institutional arrangements a caring government should have is certainly a public health system to remedy sickness and injury and to help in frail old age and disability. Thus, *a* common, sharable morality may be based on the following *political* principle justified by the first principle of normative ethics: "individuals have a right to equal concern and respect in the design and administration of the political institutions that govern them".[26] In other words, caring & respecting requires: health care policies (preventive care, primary and acute care, social services for those with disabilities etc.), basic education for all (teaching useful skills, cultivating artistic talents, giving physical training etc. and enforcing one's own sense of responsibility), public safety (protection from different kinds of harm) etc. for all vulnerable human beings. All these policies can be integrated by the concept of respectful care. In this sense, *a* common, sharable, morality may be based on egalitarian and universal norms, but capable of respecting differences at the same time. It is also the best candidate for providing the juridical foundation to guarantee respect for other basic rights such as the freedom to pursue one's ideals, life projects etc. and other fundamental liberties such as having property. Last but not least, *a* common, sharable morality guarantees mutual respect among persons,

---

[24] Daniel Engster, *The Heart of Justice*, (Oxford: Oxford University Press, 2009), 72. For an application of a care ethics in the political domain, including the global arena, see also: Virginia Held, *Ethics of Care*, (Oxford: Oxford University Press, 2006).

[25] Daniel Engster, *The Heart of Justice*, (Oxford: Oxford University Press, 2009), 76f. Regarding what is *basic* or *non-basic*, we can adopt the sufficient principle. It states that "special concern for any being B is appropriate up to the point at which B has a level of wellbeing such that B can live a life which is sufficiently good." On this point see: Roger Crisp, *Reasons & the Good*, (Oxford: Oxford University Press, 2008), 160.

[26] Ronald Dworkin, *Taking Rights Seriously*, (Cam. /Mass: Harvard University Press, 1978), 180.

limiting doctrines (for example, traditional practices, religions etc.) which are incompatible with the above mentioned moral attitude.

CHAPTER SIX

APPLYING RESPECTFUL CARE

Having sorted out the concept of respectful care, I would now like to apply it to the bioethical cases reconstructed in the previous chapters and to ask what should have been done to avoid the problems that happened. Let me first of all underline the point that the concept of respectful care refers to a particular moral *attitude* we all must have in all the domains of our lives. It leads to what is optimific, universally willable and would not be rejected by a virtuous person. As such, it is also capable of providing the right normative standard for bioethical cases. Thus, in the first section, I will go back to the stories of Baby 1, Baby 2 and Baby 3 to assess what would have been the right course of action had respectful care been taken seriously. In the second section, I will examine the role of some institutions such as (bio)ethics committees and the legal system in ensuring respectful care.

6.1 Back to the cases: Baby 1, Baby 2 and Baby 3

I would now like, in light of the concept of respectful care, to re-examine the cases we have been scrutinizing to find out what should have happened had it been applied to them. The main intention is to show how we may avoid similar problems happening again. The idea is not to pass a final judgment, but to help to understand better our practices and to avoid new mistakes. It is also important to bear in mind that this will be done from the point of view of *a* common, sharable morality, which may leave space for diverse decisions based on the values and beliefs of persons belonging to particular moral systems.

Before re-examining the cases, let me recall the main meta-ethical and normative results of the previous chapters. These were the main achievements: (i) a new moral epistemology (practical cognitivism) was put forward to solve the difficulties of intuitionist meta-ethics overcoming, in this way, most of the problems of principlism; (ii) an amended Triple Theory established a first principle for *a* common, sharable morality, namely *act under norms that are optimific, universally willable and would not be rejected by a virtuous person.* This formal metanorm has the potential to overcome most of the differences between consequentialists, deontologists and virtue ethicists. If this is the case, it is a huge development in contemporary normative ethics. More importantly for bioethical purposes, it provides an objective criterion to apply the basic norms of bioethics, which were *reduced* to caring and respecting.

There is no doubt that the above mentioned first principle is formal. It can, however, be *specified* into basic norms such as "do good, avoid evil," "respect persons" etc. Now, one may even think that these two norms can be made to *converge*. Consider this: on the one hand, if we take the non-maleficence principle as forbidding doing more harm than good and afterwards specify violating rights as a kind of harm, that is, *moral* harm, then we can run the whole gamut of which rights exist and justify them by appealing to that norm; on the other hand, if we start with the principle of respect for persons and afterwards specify kinds of harm as forms of disrespect, then we have the same result. But if we want to keep the *limiting* function of both care & respect avoiding indifference and paternalism, then we must not attempt to reduce care to respect or the other way around. It is not possible to reduce care to respect or respect to care without losing substantial contents of our moral life. To use a common way of putting it: beneficence and justice are different in kind. Besides, the formal convergence of consequentialists, deontologists and virtue ethicists under the first principle reveals a way to overcome the arbitrary and relativistic applications of the *two* basic notions of bioethics. To fill in its formal letter, we may specify either rights or kinds of harm.

I will here consider premature babies persons in the *dispositional* sense, so this is perhaps the best place to present some further reasons for asserting the principle of respect *for persons* and not just respect *for autonomy* as a basic norm of bioethics. Before presenting some reasons for doing so, let me give one more example of the ethical problems in neonatal bioethics. In his recent book *Death or Disability?* Dominic Wilkinson assumes the view that there is a hierarchy in the medical decision-making process. In his own words:

> At the top of the three is Autonomy –for competent patients we should act in accordance with their wishes. Western medical ethics has raised autonomy to a position of pre-eminence. We usually think that doctors should respect a patient's wishes even if the patient is clearly mistaken about what would be best for them, unless they are mentally ill or otherwise incompetent to make a decision. Below this principle is Substituted Judgement. For patients who are not able to express their wishes, but who were previously competent we should be guided by what

> we believe they would have wanted. This is the basis for the use of advance directives, and is one of the reasons why families are involved in decision-making for adults – they are often a good source of information about the desires and preferences of the patient. Finally, at the lowest level of the tree lies Best Interests. For patients who are incompetent and whose wishes are either unknown or unknowable (as is the case for infants and young children) we should be guided by what would be best for them.[1]

As can be seen, Wilkinson apparently assumes a moderate liberal view of medical ethics, placing autonomy in the highest place. However, when in chapter 8 of *Death or Disability?* he presents a threshold framework for decisions, we realize that, in fact, his main proposal aims essentially at setting quite narrow limits for parental discretion, which fall below what seems required by the principle of respect for persons.

We can grasp Wilkinson's proposal in two ways: first, he thinks that there is a level of impairment sufficiently severe that certain types of treatment should *not* be provided even if the parents wish it; second, and at the other end, there is a level of impairment sufficiently mild that life-sustaining treatment must continue even if parents do not want this to occur.[2] Thus, strangely enough, parents do have a say, especially because babies' and parents' interests overlap, but *only* when doctors are *uncertain* about whether treatment should be withdrawn or should continue. This proposal produces, I believe, an unbalanced relation between caring & respecting. That is to say, it still gives doctors too wide a scope for autocratic decisions leaving to the babies' parents a very narrow margin for autonomous decisions. But, according to what is required by respectful care, parents always have the right to participate in the decision-making process.

Now, one of the main reasons for keeping respect for persons instead of autonomy, understood essentially as individual self-determination, is that the latter is *one* right among others only. Moreover, respect for autonomy is not enough to balance the power between scientists/doctors and subjects/patients. Why not? Because doctors can always decide whether or not an individual is autonomous by, for instance, making an assessment of his competence for decision-making, questioning whether she has mental disorders or does not understand the information given, and so on. Now, if we keep respect for persons as the Belmont Report does and

---

[1] Dominic Wilkinson, *Death or Disability*? (Oxford: Oxford University Press, 2013), 48-9.

[2] For a better explanation of the threshold framework for decisions, see: Dominic Wilkinson, *Death or Disability*? (Oxford: Oxford University Press, 2013), 261f.

we assume that a person has several intrinsic rights such as freedom, equal treatment, satisfaction of basic needs including to be cared for, etc., then it is outside the doctor's domain to question one particular right. Finally, it becomes clearer how to hold a health professional accountable, especially, when she violates such rights.

A second reason for keeping the stronger principle of respect for persons in bioethics and not just autonomy/self-determination is that it forbids many forms of manipulative action not only in the relationship between health professionals/scientists and patients/subjects of research, but also among patients themselves.[3] For instance, it forbids collecting an organ *just* for commercial reasons. This was a famous counterexample to classical utilitarianism: kill an innocent person with healthy organs to save five patients. It is wrong to maximize utility by using persons as a mere means since everyone counts as one. Now, an autonomous individual could deliberate and decide to donate his own kidney. But if it is just to make money, it is immoral since it violates one's own integrity, one's own personhood. Thus, the principle of respect for persons is capable of forbidding such an act. It is a health professional's or scientist's duty to prevent a patient or a subject of research treating herself as a non-person. That is to say, if we consider only respect for autonomy, then health professionals may come to view patients on the basis of their goals and preferences, and, eventually, "it may lead us to disrespect persons."[4] Consequently, an exclusive focus on individual autonomy may lead to a distortion of the recognition of the person *qua* person, annihilating morality itself.

We may now recognise that the principle that protects persons and not just the simple right to autonomy, which is the basic norm in *knowing-how* to respect, is capable of justifying a set of particular *virtues* and *rules* guiding scientists and subjects, health professionals and patients: veracity, confidentiality, privacy, fidelity etc. These rules, if internalized, lead to correspondent attitudes. The principle of respect for persons can also, as we have seen, incorporate the basic idea of distributive justice: a person has the right to a fair share (equally among equals; unequally among different people). As we have seen, it is possible to reduce the principle of *distributive* justice to that of respect for persons.

---

[3] For a defence of the principle of respect for persons see my papers "Was Kant a Naturalist?" (*Studia Kantiana*. v. 14, 2013b, 141-158) and "Respect for persons" in: Darlei Dall'Agnol and Milene Tonetto (eds), *Morality and Life*, (Pisa: ETS, 2015a), 127-145.

[4] Mary Beach *et al.* "What does 'Respect' Mean?" (*Journal of General Internal Medicine*, v.22, 2007), 693.

Another reason to keep respect for *persons* and not just for autonomy/self-determination is the assumption that one person cannot autonomously decide to do harm to herself or to others. The moral norm "at least, do no harm" pre-exists the relationship between a physician and a patient in common sense morality. It is a principle regulating persons' relationships in everyday life. This basic principle is one of the main tenets of *a* common, sharable morality, universally valid, and capable of overcoming present-day relativism. In this sense, I do agree with Professor Rauscher, namely that an "ethics of respect for persons would be realist rather than idealist."[5] I argued for the realist feature of practical cognitivism in the previous chapter.

When bioethicists hold that respect for autonomy should prevail and not respect for persons, they are using the word 'autonomy' in an individualistic sense. There is, consequently, a real difference between the two principles: respect for persons and respect for autonomy. Respect for persons means something other than just respect for self-determination. Granted, self-determination is a moral right, and from the 1990s onwards, it has been also a legal right in the US, but a person is entitled to more rights than just this one. In some sense, the principle respect for persons has a bigger extension than the principle respect for autonomy: it may include, for instance, the right to health assistance. This right is not just a legal one (in Brazil it is, but not in the US). As we have seen, it is a *moral* one, so it must be enforced by a common, sharable morality, and I will return to this point below when I examine the implications of taking a newborn as a person in the dispositional sense. Thus, having recalled the main meta-ethical and normative results of the previous chapters and having stressed the importance of respect for persons, let me examine further the bioethics cases previously presented.

To start with, consider Baby 1's story again. No doubt, her wellbeing needed serious medical attention. The baby's *symptoms* of pain were clear enough: frequent grimacing, writhing, tightening her abdomen, increased agitation, decreased sleep etc. The *signs* of her condition were: the baby was medically unstable (blood pressure); most of her small intestines were dead; she had liver failure; the major arteries supplying blood to the intestines were clotted off etc. Caring for *her*, in this case, could have just meant relieving her pain if a cure was not possible. After all, caring must not be conflated with providing a cure; care is not reducible to treatment. What is clear, then, is that Baby 1 needed serious attention regarding her

[5] For a further discussion on this topic see: Frederick Rauscher, "Realism and Anti-realism in Kant's Meta-Ethics." In: Milene Tonetto *et al.* (eds.), *Investigações Kantianas I*, (Florianópolis: Funjab, 2012), p.40f.

wellbeing. As we have seen, the object of a health professional's attention is the patient's wellbeing, not only her health, and that means caring in all its mental, spiritual and physical dimensions. One could describe objectively Baby 1's heath condition, but the symptoms of suffering are subjective. One may even think that morphine has the same effect on everyone, but *this* particular patient suffering at this specific time may have different causes for her pain, and sometimes giving more morphine is not the only or even the best solution. Here caring appears to have an objective element. That is to say, health may be taken as a descriptive concept and Baby 1's health is not *necessarily* composed of what her parents in fact *wish* at a particular moment, but it constitutes what they should wish for her own wellbeing. That is why reasons to care are, in some sense, agent-neutral. But a health professional and the family may disagree about the *value* of health or even its hierarchical place in the family's axiological system. Moreover, since Baby 1's quality of life is composed of her health conditions, her psychophysical wellbeing as a functioning organism comprising many sub-systems *and* her family values (especially how they value life itself, health etc.), the conclusion is that parents must *always* have a say in the decision-making process. We must keep in mind that to care for someone respectfully means to address her wellbeing, including her health, without violating other rights.

As I already pointed out in the first chapter, Baby 1's case involves a metaphysical dispute between a scientific approach and a religious worldview. We should, however, ask whether the parents' attitude was justified in bringing religious arguments to the stage, for instance, expecting a miracle. Certainly, this is inappropriate in respectfully caring for the baby and they should have acted differently. Baby 1's parents cannot demand, based on a religious belief, to increase "care" if this implies only doing more and more harm to their daughter. To recognize this point, consider different parental reactions. In their study "Moral and Ethical Dilemmas in the Special-Care Nursery," Duff and Campbell summed up a variety of different views that knowledgeable parents (such as physicians, nurses, lawyers) could have about babies in such circumstances:

> Some thought their child had a right to die since he could not live well or effectively. Others thought that society should pay the costs of care that may be so destructive to the family economy. Often, too, the parent's or siblings' rights to relief from the seemingly pointless, crushing burdens

> were important considerations. It seemed right to yield to parent wishes in several cases as physicians have done for generations.[6]

The authors report a case of an infant with Down syndrome and intestinal atresia, which was not treated because his parents thought that the surgery was wrong for their baby and themselves. One may hold that a right to die is just part of the right to life. But the Baby 1 case is different since the parents were arguing for and even requesting –in fact, demanding– *more* care and they felt disrespected in their right to decide. One may wonder why people have different reactions and take different attitudes and decisions. The answer lies in pluralism: a different family could react differently, that is to say, let Baby 1 go and focus on the possibility of a new baby later. Thus, it seems clear that conflicting moral frameworks, either based on naturalist/scientific or supranaturalist/religious views of the world, played a role in the deliberation about what to do in this case.

To understand better this point, it is crucial not to forget that Baby 1 was in a very special institution, that is, in a medical school. One may ask then what is the main role of such institutions. What is the function of teaching hospitals such as the ones involved in the Baby 1 and Baby 2 cases? Certainly, one mission of such institutions is to advance *scientific knowledge* and not only to treat patients. A Catholic hospital might have different goals and would probably forgo treatment for Baby 1 including nutrition. That is why Baby 1's story is a bioethical case and not only a problem for medical ethics. Thus, one may wonder whether some sort of scientific "curiosity" was not underlying the keeping of Baby 1 alive for so long. What could "school professionals" in their dual role as scientists and as doctors learn from this case? Was Baby 1 just "teaching material" as the parents thought? Certainly, that would be completely immoral, that is, a form of disrespect for persons.

There is no doubt that teaching hospitals are a very special kind of institution. They have to train new doctors. That is to say, residents get their care skills by helping and essentially by practicing. They learn by doing and only practice makes perfect. Recalling practical cognitivism, they need to learn their *knowings-how*: how to care; how to treat; how to respect patients' rights etc. In this context, the need for a new moral epistemology makes plain sense, and has the potential to overcome the

---

[6] Raymond Duff and Campbell, A. G. M. "Moral and Ethical Dilemmas in the Special-Care Nursery" in: Nancy Jecker *et al.* (eds.), *Bioethics*, (Sudbury: Jones and Bartlett Publishers, 1997), 63.

problems of principlism and other bioethical theories.[7] Some need also to learn *how* to increase scientific knowledge. This generates all sorts of conflicts, especially between increasing the patient's wellbeing and the need to make scientific progress. These conflicts need to be solved by placing respectful care above anything else, for instance, above personal professional interests such as the pressure to publish more papers just to be recognized in the scientific community.

I would now like to mention some legal directives the US has adopted regarding scientific experimentation on humans since the story of Baby 1 happened in that country. The American Medical Association (AMA) *Ethics Guidelines Regarding Clinical Investigation* explicitly allows for experimentation on minors. One of the guidelines prescribes that minors or mentally incompetent persons may be used as subjects in clinical investigation only if:

i) the nature of the investigation is such that mentally competent adults would not be suitable subjects;
ii) consent, in writing, is given by a legally authorized representative of the subject under circumstances in which informed and prudent adults would reasonably be expected to volunteer themselves or their children as subjects.

Is there then evidence that Baby 1 was used "merely as a means", that is, just as an *object* of scientific research? In the first case, the parents *did*, according to their blog, feel that their child was being treated as a kind of "lab assignment." Suppose then that the U. of A., having not yet done a small intestine transplant, or just willing to do it for *teaching* purposes, considered undertaking a transplant procedure despite the fact that the intestine was dead. This could also be the case with Baby 2: her surgery could be just *experimental*, the first of its kind for a particular surgeon using a new drug. Given the above guidelines, it seems clear that the parents' consent would be sufficient to authorize children to be used as subjects in scientific experimentation. Is this ethical?

It is certainly controversial. Many bioethicists hold that children cannot ever be subject to experiments if they are not potential beneficiaries. For one, in his book *The Patient as Person*, Paul Ramsey sorted out the presuppositions and implications of an ethics of consent in medicine for

---

[7] In this sense, it is very easy to commit mistakes. For instance, NEC in the Baby 1 case could be an iatrogenic illness caused by incorrect feeding. For a discussion on iatrogenic illness see: Virginia Sharpe and Alan Faden, *Medical Harm*, (Cambridge: Cambridge University Press, 1998).

children. In the first chapter "Consent as a Canon of Loyalty with Special Reference to Children in Medical Investigations," Ramsey argued that children, who cannot give mature and informed consent,

> … should not be made the subjects of medical experimentation unless, other remedies having failed to relieve their grave illness, it is reasonable to believe that the administration of a drug as yet untested or insufficiently tested on human beings, or the performance of an untried operation, may further *the patient's own recovery*.[8]

This general rule for physician-investigators sets a clear limit for dealing with subject experimentations: where there is no possible benefit for the child's own recovery, an infant is not to be made a mere object in medical experimentation for some ulterior good. Otherwise, the patient will be disrespected. We must always remember that respecting a person is intrinsically valuing her, and that caring for a vulnerable being for her own sake is an instantiation of the very same attitude. Ramsey characterizes experimenting on children in a way that is not related to them as "a sanitized form of barbarism."[9] He goes on to maintain that no parent *should* consent to any experiment upon children with no relation to their possible treatment. To consent is to treat a child as not a child, but as if she were an adult person who could consent. Ramsey allows for just one exception to his general rule: epidemic conditions. He mentions as an example Dr. Salk, who tried his polio vaccine on himself and his own children first and then tested it on selected children since it involved some risk that the disease might be contracted from the vaccine itself.

We may then conclude that the health team working on Baby 1's case at the U. of A., as a teaching facility, acted rightly by not explicitly transforming the patient into a mere object of scientific experiences. That would be against the idea of intrinsically valuing the patient. Another right decision was not to increase care if that meant only doing more harm to Baby 1. We must keep in mind that it is a hinge-practical proposition not to cause more harm than benefit. But since the decision to give nutrition may be considered a parental one, the health team should not have withdrawn life-sustaining measures in the first place without the *explicit* authorization of the parents. Unfortunately, there are more wrongs than rights in the Baby 1 case: i) the U. of A. did not explain in clear language

---

[8] Paul Ramsey, *The Patient as Person*, (New Haven/London: Yale University Press, 1977), 11-2.

[9] Paul Ramsey, *The Patient as Person*, (New Haven/London: Yale University Press, 1977), 12.

the difference between treatment and palliative care; that is to say, the conditions of informed consent were not met and thus the hospital was not authorized to do anything in the name of the parents; ii) the ethics committee acted in an unethical way by not allowing for a transfer, that is, by not permitting Baby 1 to have a *real second opinion*; iii) the health team obfuscated the family's perception about what they could do because some of the health professionals were saying that the committee had decided and that they couldn't do anything; iv) society and the hospital as a public institution acted unfairly by not giving the baby a real chance since the insurance did not cover everything Baby 1 needed; v) the court acted in an unconstitutional way by not providing a "speedy decision"; vi) the family did not think about the harm they could be doing to their baby by trying extraordinary means. Now, balancing the rights and wrongs in this case, it is evident that there were more immoral actions. That is to say, respect was not in place and care was absent. This is the opposite to what a common, sharable morality, based on respectful care, requires.

Recalling the results of section 4.2 on killing or letting die, I would like now to point out that, if Baby 1 had had different parents, they could have chosen a different outcome. One could, for instance, ask for a lethal injection instead of letting the baby die or keeping her alive at any cost. To the question "Who would do it?" I have a simple answer: the same people who decide "to let die."[10] This solution is compatible with what is required by *a* common, sharable morality based on respectful care. Thus, I believe that society must put into place several institutional arrangements to provide for active non-voluntary euthanasia for those parents who want it for babies in similar conditions. As I have pointed out elsewhere (2012c), these conditions are:

i) the futility of the treatment must be assured by two medical teams (unfortunately, this was not the case in the Baby 1 story);
ii) the consent is really obtained in a free and informed way (Baby 1's parents did not understand the implications of "palliative care only", so they did not really consent);
iii) the ethics committee must review the case giving the "go ahead";
iv) the judiciary or a prosecutor, in society's name, provides the final authorization.

[10] If we want to preserve medicine's goals since "doctors must not kill," then the solution should be similar to the death penalty case, which in the US is legal anyway. Again, medicine's *telos* may be not only curing, but relieving pain and suffering too.

Hopefully, these and other necessary institutional arrangements will make it possible to provide both care & respect, that is, respectful care in a proper way.

Baby 1's parents, however, did not want this to happen to their daughter. Then, we could adopt Texas's solution giving them one week to find another facility willing to treat their baby. As I said previously, perhaps a Catholic hospital would have treated Baby 1. In the next section, I will examine in a more detailed way some necessary institutions for caring respectfully, especially the roles of ethics committees.

Before discussing the case of Baby 2, let me here point out that we should at this point be crystal clear on the differences between active and passive euthanasia. What makes the former permissible is parents' permission. Thus, perhaps this is also the right place to say that some distinctions on this subject are not very helpful. It is common among some Brazilian bioethicists to discriminate between orthotanasia and dysthanasia. Orthotanasia means "right death" (from the Greek *ortos* and *thanatos*). It is defined as not prolonging artificially the death process beyond the natural process. Orthotanasia is, however, an idealized concept bioethicists invented because they think that euthanasia is always an anticipation of death. But this is not necessarily so. Thus, in the end, orthotanasia seems to be just a synonym for passive euthanasia. Now, dysthanasia (from the Greek *dys*, difficult, bad) is the undue prolonging of life by artificial means in a person who could not otherwise survive. Dysthanasia is a bad death because it prolongs patients' biological life without considering their quality of life. To avoid that, we must choose either active or passive euthanasia. Thus, we must bear in mind that different parents would choose divergent courses of action regarding cases such as Baby 1's and *a* common, sharable morality must justify institutional arrangements to meet different outcomes: either active or passive euthanasia.

Regarding Baby 2, there was a first moment when the baby was left to die because of her extreme prematurity. This was understandable given her low APGAR score and other data available at that time. But the health professionals did the right thing given the signs the patient showed afterwards, and the decision to treat her shows that respectful care was in place. Moreover, the surgical intervention was recommended from a medical point of view and it was successful. The quality of life Baby 2 has today is a proof of how much neonatalogy, based on sound bioethical norms and the right attitude, is doing for us.

Baby 2's life was saved using taxpayers' resources through the Brazilian SUS, a public and universal health system. This exemplifies what is required by respectful care, especially what is a sound application of principles of justice. In the case of Baby 1, issues relating to resources were also an ethical problem. The parents' health insurance was a major cause of not providing the best possible care. In a universal health system, Baby 1 would perhaps have been better off. In the Baby 3 case, she was in a similar system (NHS), but she didn't receive the best possible care to answer her basic needs in a midwife-led maternity unit. Again, we need to discuss the best institutional and social arrangements necessary to satisfy the requirements of respectful care. In the Baby 2 case, the "informed consent form" was not even signed by the parents and that is something an ethics committee could be in charge of enforcing. Baby 2's surgery was in some sense also experimental ('experimental' doesn't mean here necessarily innovative or aimed at making scientific or technological progress). But it was a clear mistake in Baby 2's case not to give the appropriate attention to informed consent for invasive procedures. This was a concrete form of disrespect. Can we say that this is *relative* to Brazilian medical culture and that in the US it would not have happened? It is reasonable to assume, *pace* most Brazilian bioethicists who support a "hard bioethics" of intervention and argue that autonomy fits only the North American context, that obtaining consent is a universal requirement for respecting persons. Thus, cultural differences do not justify ethical relativism. As can be seen, ethical relativism does not seem true even if there is no *the* unique moral system and we are bound to accept some degree of value pluralism. A common, sharable morality is a condition to make such pluralism reasonable warranting peaceful co-existence, all forms of cooperation etc., and allowing space for personal decisions.

Regarding Baby 3, there is little doubt that respectful care was absent. Thus, a universal health system is not sufficient for respectful care. As became clear, Baby 3's "care" was disrespectful in many ways, for example, a second opinion should have been sought, the baby should not have been delivered in a midwife unit etc. I believe that Baby 3 died an avoidable and wrongful death. Apparently, both parents and midwife professionals did not care for the *baby's own sake*. That is to say, this case clearly shows a lack of respect as an expression of an intrinsic valuation, that is, of *not* knowing-how professionals ought to behave for the patient's own sake. As the health ombudsman report now reveals, the baby's records are of a poor standard and even inaccurate in some places. There is no doubt that the midwife missed key signs that *the baby* was unwell, so she did not care for *the patient's own sake.* If we are to avoid such cases occurring again, we have not only to improve the material and scientific conditions to provide proper care, but we need also to add a moral dimension to caring: delivering it respectfully.

As I argued in the last chapter, respectful care requires not only good intentions or nice feelings such as sympathy or even empathy or compassion, but also real material conditions to benefit a vulnerable individual at risk of losing her life. Baby 3's death could have been avoided. I am not saying that generally midwives are not caring professionals or that a midwifery unit is not the right place for a caring decision. All I wanted to do was to illustrate what the concept of respectful care requires. The attention needed to improve a patient's wellbeing, to restore her health or simply to protect her from further harm must be accompanied by effective knowledge, both scientifically and morally speaking, and by material conditions. There are many mistakes that care is subjected to. Technical errors, for instance in diagnosis, are not the only ones that may occur. Moral failure may also be the case. The conclusion cannot be other: poor care, as provided in the Baby 3 case, is very disrespectful indeed.

It is worth underlining the fact that in the Baby 1, Baby 2 and Baby 3 stories, as in any case indeed, respectful care *must* always be provided. It is required by the first principle of normative ethics spelt out in the previous chapter: it is optimific, universally willable and would not be rejected by a virtuous person.

Now, premature infants are certainly not autonomous beings and they cannot consent or choose anything. They are, however, persons in a dispositional sense. Thus, there are disrespectful "caring" actions, which are prohibited by a common, sharable morality, for instance, doing transplants without the parents' consent. There is no way back and informed consent must always be obtained in bioethical experiments using human subjects for scientific research. This means that the person involved should have the capacity to give consent; should be so situated as to be able to exercise free power of choice, without the intervention of any element of force, fraud, deceit, duress, overreaching, or other ulterior form of constraint or coercion; and should have sufficient knowledge and comprehension of the elements of the subject matter involved as to enable her to make a discerning and enlightened decision. As we have seen, under the Belmont Report's principles, the babies were protected, but under the transformations of this approach carried out by Beauchamp and Childress this is not clearly so. Now, the principle of substituted judgment says that the surrogate decision-maker should choose as the individual would choose for herself if she could; or if the surrogate decision-maker cannot know how an individual would decide, then she needs to take into account the patient's best interests. Better to bear in mind all the rights a person has in deciding for babies such as Baby 1, Baby 2, Baby 3 and … any premature baby indeed.

To finish this section, I would like to provide a clear advantage of using a single concept such as respectful care in analysing bioethical cases. The reason is straightforward: for theoretical and practical *simplicity*. Now, in manuals one may find a multiplicity of guidelines that should be used to educate new neonatal caregivers. For instance, in the book *Comprehensive Neonatal Care*, the authors synthesized, based on the American Academy of Paediatrics (AAP, 2000), the following core principles for caring for patients (new-borns and infants):[11]

- Respecting the dignity of both child and caregiver.
- Being sensitive to and respectful of the family's wishes.
- Using the most appropriative measures that are consistent with the family's choices.
- Encompassing alleviation of pain and other physical symptoms.
- Assessing and managing psychologic, social, and spiritual/religious problems.
- Ensuring continuity of care (the child should be able to continue to be cared for, if so desired, by his/her primary care and specialist providers).
- Providing access to any therapy that may realistically be expected to improve the child's quality of life, including alternative or non-traditional treatments.
- Providing access to palliative care and hospice care.
- Respecting the right to refuse treatment that may prolong suffering of life.
- Respecting the physician's professional responsibility to discontinue some treatments when appropriate, with consideration for both child and family's preferences.
- Promoting clinical evidence-based research on providing care at the end of life.

Note how many times care & respect appears in the above guidelines. In fact, each norm sorts out actions which are expressions of looking after respectfully a vulnerable being. Therefore, for simplicity's sake, we could just speak in terms of *respectful care*. This is the single attitude that must be enforced in *a* common, sharable morality. *Simplifying all norms into a*

[11] Kenner, C. and Lott, J. W., *Comprehensive Neonatal Care*, (St. Louis/Missouri: Saunders, 2007), 512.

single concept referring to an attitude is one of the most important results of the present work.

In the next section, I will discuss the role of some institutional arrangements in providing respectful care, especially ethics committees and the legal system. The intention is to show that respectful care needs proper social and political conditions to flourish.

6.2 The roles of (bio)ethics committees

In this section, I will examine the responsibilities some institutions have in taking decisions on matters of life and death and, particularly, discuss the roles of (bio)ethics committees in defining what to do in cases like the ones we have been examining. The main objective is to show that different agents have diverse grounds for their choices and, therefore, we must be crystal clear on what each person can and must take a decision on. As we will see, a crucial role (bio)ethics committees must have is to secure that respectful care is always in place.

It seems clear that the decision-making process sometimes involves many persons in most bioethical cases. To establish the roles each has, we may follow the contributions of Shannon, who identifies the following moments in the decision-making process: (i) the medical dimensions of the case; (ii) the context of the decision and (iii) the decision-making itself.[12] Now, regarding the decision-making process, he raises two main questions: *Who decides*? and, perhaps more importantly, *On what basis*?

On the question *Who decides*? there are four possibilities: the parents, the health team, society or the ethics committees. The answer must take into consideration the results of the previous chapters, especially that philosophy understood as knowing-how to live well leads to value pluralism, which does not mean relativism since it is only possible under the necessary condition of *a* common, sharable morality. Now, the parents are the persons who planned to have the child and, consequently, have full responsibility for nurturing her. Physicians have skills, knowledge and experience and are committed to preserving life. Ethics committees need to be open and take decisions not hidden under the guise of the supposedly technical features of the case only. Society as a whole, manly represented by the courts of law, must guarantee impartiality and fairness in the whole process.

---

[12] Thomas Shannon, *An Introduction to Bioethics*, (New York: Paulist Press, 1997), 95.

The bioethical cases we have been discussing show that parents are responsible for making decisions for their children. Now, if there is a conflict with the medical team's recommendations, then the (bio)ethics committee is the first place to appeal. This, of course, does not mean that an ethics committee has a decision-making role. Given the pluralistic character grounded by *a* common, sharable morality, it seems clear that patients themselves are normally the best candidates to have this prerogative. The ethics committee may try to solve the conflict between the parts only. Finally, if the ethics committee is unable to dissolve the conflict, which reveals itself as persistent because of opposing values and incompatible beliefs, then the court is the place for a final decision.

On the question *On what basis?* there are three standards: medical, quality of life and substituted judgment. Here, the fundamental medical issues are: is this condition treatable? Is it manageable? Is it reversible? Can the patient benefit? The quality of life standard relates to the question that while physical life is a value, it may not be the ultimate value for every person. Finally, the substituted judgment is an attempt to put oneself in the position of the child and make the decision one thinks the child would make if she knew what the decision makers know. As we have seen, a cure may not always be possible. Care, especially real palliative care, is *always* required in such cases if there is no treatment available, regardless of further decisions and procedures in taking life.

I will from now on argue that (bio)ethics committees have a fundamental role, namely *to secure that the conditions for caring & respecting are always met*, but have no explicit decision-making function. One of the main ideas for a (bio)ethics committee is that of reconciling divergent views (conflicts between parents and health professionals) about the best course of action to be taken helping them to resolve ethical doubts. Such committees are an attempt to provide a forum for ethical decisions given pluralism and the moral disagreement it generates. If this fails, then the legal system, based on the requirements of *a* common, sharable morality has the last word on what must be done.

Bearing these considerations in mind, let me go back to our cases and ask what the committee could have done. Consider what the Paediatrics Ethics Committee of the U. of A. decided regarding the case of Baby 1:

> Since physicians have determined that the patient's condition is terminal and incurable, further medical interventions other than comfort measures are futile and transfer to another facility does not serve the best interests of this child. Furthermore, since continued medical interventions offer no reasonable medical benefit to the patient and such interventions serve only to postpone the moment of death, the treatment team is under no moral

> obligation to continue life-sustaining treatment. *The parent's right to seek a second opinion has been met.* Since it has been determined that no additional interventions can be offered to this child, there is no benefit in transferring her to another facility (italics added).

Granted, establishing whether a patient has an incurable condition and whether she is terminal is a purely medical prerogative (remembering, though, that medicine is not an exact science), but the decision not to transfer to another facility is incompatible with the insistence that the right to have a *real* second opinion was respected. Thus, it seems that care & respect were not really provided in a proper, balanced way in this case.

The official statement from the U. of A. says that they met with the parents and the second opinion was given, but Baby 1's parents disagreed. On the family's blog (09/14) one can read: "No it has not been met! We can't get an unbiased assessment of our child because of the committee meeting!" Now, the problem is not only whether or not the right to the second opinion was met. The problem is that the U. of A. *should not* have decided not to allow a transfer. This is, certainly, not a matter an ethics committee should decide upon. Why then didn't the ethics committee allow a transfer?

Let me point out that (bio)ethics committees are also supposed to be "the impartial judges" when a conflict between a patient's preferences and the health team arises. An ethics committee shares responsibility for the axiological dimensions of the case and normally comprises professionals from interdisciplinary backgrounds. It cannot have any punitive function whatsoever and must above all avoid abusive actions. Thus, in no circumstance may an ethics committee push the institutional view onto the patient/subject of scientific research. Actual ethics committees may, however, have a lot of problems which impair rather than improve decisions: members may pressure patients to reach a consensus; they may avoid controversial issues; underestimate risks etc. But they cannot and must never *deny* the patient's right to leave the hospital whenever she wants to seek a second opinion. They cannot deny in any circumstance a transfer and in Baby 1's case the *crux of the matter* is that she had in fact no real second opinion because of the committee's decision. It is difficult not to arrive at the conclusion that the U. of A.'s ethics committee acted unethically. If care & respect, when balanced in the proper way, mean basically improving the welfare of vulnerable beings *without* violating other rights, then clearly the ethics committee at the U. of A. did not secure these fundamental moral elements in its practices. On the contrary, it decided against what *respectful care* prescribes.

This remark brings us to the question of the *composition* and not only the *roles* of ethics committees in clinical and hospital contexts. Since the New Jersey Supreme Court, after analysing the case of Karen Quinlan, ordered the creation of ethics committees in hospitals 40 years ago, their role has been widely discussed. By the 1980s, almost every hospital in the US had an ethics committee. Many commentators ask whether such committees can have an active decision-making role or only other functions such as helping to clarify ethically ambiguous cases, confirming prognoses, etc.

On this particular point, Robert Veatch correctly endorses functions such as developing and recommending ethics-related policies, advising, etc., but rules out decisions.[13] According to him, there are four main possible functions:

i) To review cases to confirm the responsible physician's diagnosis and prognosis of a patient's medical condition;
ii) To provide a forum for discussing broader social and ethical concerns raised by a particular case and, in so doing, to teach professional staff how to identify, frame, and resolve ethics problems;
iii) To formulate policy and guidelines regarding such decisions;
iv) To review decisions made by other professionals about the treatment of specific patients or make such decisions themselves.

The last role is ambiguous and brings in fact two conflicting policies: whether the committee has only an *advisory* function or whether it has a *decisionary* role.

The best role a (bio)ethics committee has is to provide a forum for discussion of ethical conflicts. It may help with difficult decisions because the best medical care requires not only medical skills, but sound moral judgment based on respectful care. We need such forums because caring for sick newborn infants may raise concerns about the appropriateness of the management in relation to the expected outcome. The committee's main purpose is to offer help and guidance on moral and ethical questions, such as: should treatment be started or stopped? How much should a child be told about his or her disease? Is the promise of treatment worth the suffering it may cause? What is the best thing to do when we must face the end of life? It is almost unnecessary to recall that in a forum of discussion,

[13] Robert Veatch, "Hospital Ethics Committees: is there a role?" in: Nancy Jecker, *et al.* (eds), *Bioethics*, (Boston: Jones and Bartlett Publishers. 2007), 226-231.

communication is paramount. In the Baby 1 case, however, communication broke down at a certain point and this should not have happened. Thus, a (bio)ethics committee may, for instance, have an *educational* role promoting communicative skills among the health team members.

Regarding the composition of (bio)ethics committees, they, in general, comprise members of the medical, nursing, social and pastoral hospital staff and may include an attorney and an ethicist. It seems fair enough to ask: what about a place for the patient's voice? Her absence may compromise particular decisions. Many ethicists have called attention to threats to the optimal functioning of the ethics committees. For instance, Bernard Lo gives several examples where things can go wrong: imprecise goals, restricted access and groupthink.[14] The author is really concerned with whether ethics committees are ethical since the goals and procedures of some committees may conflict with established principles and, I would add, with respectful care. For instance, a hospital administrator may suggest that the ethics committee should be used as a public relations tool for justifying unpopular decisions to discontinue unprofitable services or to discontinue life-support in many cases. This is, certainly, unethical when considered from the point of view of a common, sharable morality since it goes against the transparency required by a public system.

It seems clear, given that bioethics is a multidisciplinary field of knowledge, that committees must contain a full-time ethicist, physicians, nurses, social workers, a priest/clergy, a hospital lawyer and, in any meeting discussing a patient's interest, someone to represent her. Thus, the composition cannot have a majority, for instance, of physicians since they do not reassure patients that their wishes and interests are represented. Moreover, they may overemphasize the importance of clinical facts. In this sense, nurses are also vital: they raise overlooked issues, present new information, express the viewpoints of families, etc. Bernard Lo points out that some committees do not allow their recommendations to be reviewed, reducing the liability of individual committee members by keeping records from being discoverable, that is, from being compelled in civil suits and concludes: "such apparent secrecy may evoke the suspicion that the committee is more concerned with protecting physicians, the hospital, or itself than with helping patients."[15] This is really a fundamental point. In the Baby 1 story, the second meeting, the one that decided that the patient

[14] Bernard Lo, "Behind Closed Doors" in: Nancy Jecker *et al.* (eds.), *Bioethics*, (Boston: Jones and Bartlett Publishers. 2007), 236-244.

[15] Bernard Lo, "Behind Closed Doors" in: Nancy Jecker *et al.* (eds.), *Bioethics*, (Boston: Jones and Bartlett Publishers. 2007), 239.

should not be transferred to a different hospital, was conducted by phone. Amazingly enough, that was even acknowledged by the defendants before the court, as we saw above. That is very disrespectful indeed since a "shared responsibility" may lead to unaccountability. It diffuses liability. Consequently, I would like to propose that an *ombudsman* should be part of an ethics committee to avoid it degenerating into a mere instrument of a hospital's interests or those of the medical class. Whenever there is an obfuscation of the ethics committee's roles, for instance, in providing respectful care, the ombudsman should intervene in society's name.

We may conclude then that the main role an ethics committee has is to guarantee that *care & respect* are provided in a balanced way. That means that it can *re*-discuss the diagnosis and prognosis of a patient's medical condition, but the main focus should be on whether the patient's values and rights are in fact met. In this sense, it may, for instance, review the informed consent process. We must here remember that in the Baby 2 case the form was not signed and that this is simply unacceptable. It must also guarantee that the right to a second opinion is in fact respected. Again, we must recall that this was not guaranteed in the Baby 1 or Baby 3 cases, and that this is unacceptable too. The ethics committee must secure that all the other rights are guaranteed. In no circumstance may it deny treatment or disrespect a patient's rights. This is required by *respectful* care. If legal rights are violated, then the court is the place to appeal.

The courts normally respect ethics committees' recommendations, but in the case of Baby 1 the legal system cannot regard it as its own substitute. As we have seen, proceedings were not fair. Despite the fact that the judicial system may be too slow for clinical decisions and that a court's decision may contribute to polarizing physicians, patients and families, it seems clear that the ethics committee must not be taken as a substitute for the legal system. One can then wonder what kind of role the legal system could play in cases like Baby 1's story. Could the court order, for instance, increased care?

To answer this question properly, I need to state and justify a basic principle of the law. Briefly speaking, it says that *all persons are to be governed by a fair system of public rules specifying rights and obligations expressing the common will and applied in litigating cases by impartial judges in fair trials*. There are "political" and "juridical" elements in this principle, which need to be sorted out, but unfortunately I cannot do this here. There is no doubt, however, that this principle can be justified by an appeal to the first principle of ethics. This means basically that a law cannot exist obligating doctors to do more harm than benefit (one of our hinge- practical propositions). Since this norm is not optimific, it will not be universally willable and would not be the one subscribed to by a virtuous person. We may conclude, therefore, that the court could order increased care only to allow an immediate transfer to a different institution, but not to try to save Baby 1's life. In order to do that, the court could overrule the ethics committee's decision not to allow for a transfer, thus preserving the right to a second opinion.

The roles of the main players in the cases we have been discussing can thus be summarized in the following way: the parents decide to take the babies to the hospital and to accept or refuse offered treatment on the basis of the patients' needs and their personal values; the health teams decide on curing or not treating the patients based on medical facts and medical ethics; the (bio)ethics committees have no decision-taking role, but they can review the cases based on scientific facts and the rights/obligations of those involved making recommendations on how best to achieve respectful care. Finally, the courts guarantee legal rights for society as a whole.

Having presented the concept of respectful care and illustrated how it may work in practice, I would like now to discuss some issues related to *general* bioethics. In the last five chapters, I have been presenting a new moral epistemology for *special* (clinical and academic) bioethics only, which gave support for the concept of respectful care. We need to consider now its connections with global and holistic bioethics.

CHAPTER SEVEN

BACK TO THE FUTURE

In this last chapter, I will return to the idea that bioethics was originally meant to be a new kind of wisdom, a bridge to the future. To distinguish that idea, I used the expression "philosophical bioethics" in the first chapter, so as not to reduce bioethics to biomedical ethics. I will now discuss some problems belonging to both global and holistic bioethics. To avoid misunderstandings, one must remember that I will use 'holistic bioethics' to refer to concerns towards life as a whole, including non-human animals and the environment and 'global bioethics' to refer to international bioethical issues only. To start with, I will, in the first section, briefly examine some issues relating to future developments of science and technology, especially the construction of artificial agents either to kill or to care for vulnerable beings. This is, of course, just an illustration of some global bioethical issues. In the second section, I will go back to the original use of 'bioethics' as a general attitude towards life as a whole. I will especially examine some issues that concern us all and, consequently, must be part of *a* common, sharable morality, for instance *caring for* our environment, *caring for* non-human lifeforms etc. As I argued in chapter 1, the way to integrate special bioethics with global bioethics and holistic bioethics is through the idea of a *philosophical* bioethics.

7.1 Brave new globe: caring or killer robots?

In order to make sense of the idea of a philosophical bioethics, it is necessary to show how wisdom can guide our lives, particularly our actions and practices in biomedical contexts. In this section, I will then examine the thesis that philosophy is, as some important scientists believe, dead, arguing that this is not the case. Thus, I will examine how philosophy can, if understood as *pursuit of wisdom*, save us from a special kind of threat, namely from bad uses of artificial intelligence (AI). To illustrate, I will maintain that we should stop constructing killer robots and focus more on *caring* robots instead.

Let me start by saying that *a* common, sharable morality must, when applied globally, be capable of looking for the solutions to many current bioethical problems, that is, it must show the ways we should care more for our home helping to solve the environmental crisis, world poverty, most permanent violent conflicts, etc. To examine all these issues goes beyond the limits of this book, but I will illustrate how philosophical bioethics may help us in discussing one particular issue, which affects us all.[1] We must, however, keep in mind that *a* common, *sharable* morality is, after establishing what is communal to all human individuals, also capable of making room for differences in lifestyles, cultures, ways of thinking etc. and, consequently, justifying personal projects and different attitudes regarding some practical matters of everyday life. That is to say, *a* common, sharable morality, based on an agnostic ontology and pluralism, makes room for anyone to freely decide not only how best to act and live to achieve their projects, but may also provide some assistance in dying for those who are terminally ill and willing to do so, as I argued in the previous chapter. These policies must be applied globally, changing many existing national laws.

It is also crucial not to forget that some problems in special bioethics (e.g., clinical, neonatal bioethical issues) are closely linked to global ones: an extreme preemie may already come into the world affected by global factors such as the economic problems of her parents, a polluted environment, global warming etc. A pregnant woman living a very stressful life, working many hours under pressure, is more likely to have premature babies.[2] Moreover, a healthy person cannot live a good life in an unhealthy milieu: clean air and water are conditions for the wellbeing of *all* humans. They are basic needs we all must have met. We should, therefore, deepen our analysis looking for the bioethical conditions of life as a whole. As Potter knew, we are jeopardizing our existence. We need to redirect science and technology. This can be done by a philosophical bioethics based on wisdom.

Stephen Hawking has recently made two strong declarations, namely (i) that philosophy is dead; and (ii) that artificial intelligence could spell the end of the human race. I wonder whether there is a close connection between the two. In fact, I believe that the second will be true only if the first proves to be. But philosophy is not, as I hopefully will show now,

---

[1] For an introduction to global ethical issues, including a chapter on global bioethics see: Heather Widdows, *Global Ethics*, (Durham: Acumen, 2011), 200f.

[2] For a discussion on the causes of prematurity see: John Lantos and Diane Lauderdale, *Preterm Babies, Fetal Patients and Childbearing Choices*, (Cam/Mass.: The MIT Press, 2015).

dead and it may undoubtedly help us to prevent the catastrophic consequences of misusing science and technology. Thus, I will argue that it is through the enhancement of our *wisdom* that we can hope to avoid AI causing the end of mankind.

The first statement by Professor Hawking was made in the context of arguing that the nature of the universe could not be resolved without hard empirical data such as that provided by the Large Hadron Collider, the largest and most powerful particle collider in activity. This may well be the case, despite the fact that it may involve metaphysical issues too. He then went on to explain "Most of us don't worry about these questions most of the time. But almost all of us must sometimes wonder: Why are we here? Where do we come from? Traditionally, these are questions for philosophy, but philosophy is dead."[3] He finally concluded: "Philosophers have not kept up with modern developments in science. Particularly physics." It is difficult to see exactly what Professor Hawking meant, but he seems to subscribe to the dominant naturalist view, which asserts that scientific research and philosophical investigations are just *continuous* theoretical activities. This implies also that we could solve philosophical problems through scientific means. Despite the fact that this is a respectable view and that there is a grain of truth in it, I believe also that it misrepresents the real nature of philosophy, which has more to do with *wisdom* and not only with *scientific knowledge* about facts. Aristotle made it clear in his *Nicomachean Ethics* that philosophy was born as love of *sophia* (wisdom) not of *episteme* (scientific knowledge) or *techne* (art).[4] Thus, as it was a distortion in medieval times to make philosophy a slave of theology, it is a modern misrepresentation to reduce it to science, particularly to physics. Now, since wisdom is always needed by any person in any society, philosophy is alive and doing well indeed. This explains why Professor Hawking might also be wrong about his second prophetic statement. Philosophy is capable of showing how we can, if we are truly wise, avoid artificial intelligence causing the end of humanity. That is to say, we need *to enhance* our wisdom not artificial intelligence only.

It is crucial to recognize that philosophy has above all to do with wisdom and not with mere knowledge or intelligence. Most scientific knowledge is used to increase human wellbeing, but it can also be used to kill, to destroy the environment etc. Bioethics and other areas of practical

---

3 http://www.telegraph.co.uk/technology/google/8520033/Stephen-Hawking-tells-Google-philosophy-is-dead.html

4 Aristotle, *Nicomachean Ethics*, (Cambridge: Cambridge University Press, 2014), Book 6.

ethics were born precisely as a response to the threat posed by a positivistic understanding of the sciences and their technological misapplications. As we saw in the first chapter, Potter and many others have argued that we need *a new wisdom*, that is, the knowledge of *how to* use scientific data.[5] Thus, despite the fact that what wisdom is is open to further discussion, it seems clear that it has an irreducible practical component in guiding actions in order to live well. Many philosophers subscribe to a hybrid approach to wisdom, defining it as "knowing-how to live well." Thus, scientific knowledge is a necessary condition for wisdom so defined, but it is not a sufficient one. Further reflection on what constitutes a *good life* is also needed, and physics as a natural science has almost nothing to say on this particular point. It is here that philosophy, social sciences, ethics, that is, the humanities in general, find their *raison d'être*: to discuss the ends of our political actions, the fair basis of our legislations, the uses and misuses of scientific knowledge, what constitutes our wellbeing and so on and so forth. If the issue were to blame each other, we could say that physicists such as Hawking "have not kept up with modern developments in philosophy, particularly ethics." That is to say, Hawking's naturalism may provide answers for the fundamental questions he raises, but they would have metaphysical assumptions not shared by other persons with a different worldview. Thus, it is philosophy understood as love of wisdom that can remind us of the limits of scientific knowledge opening the way to more pluralist approaches to the world and particularly to the good life. Consequently, despite Hawking's apparent physicalism, we still need philosophical wisdom to guide us on all these issues, especially how to use scientific knowledge to live better.

I cannot sort out a complete account of wisdom here, but for my present purposes I would like to underline a significant difference between wisdom and intelligence, especially the artificial one. Again, what intelligence is is open to further discussion, but we must distinguish between a mere witty or smart person, who for instance is very skilful indeed in calculating means to achieve ends without wondering whether they are the right goals, and a wise person who is well experienced in deliberating about what is constitutive of the good life. In order to aim for the proper ends, again as Aristotle reminded us, moral virtues are essential, not only theoretical knowledge. Now, the so called "artificial intelligence" is mostly calculative reasoning based on algorithms, a very limited kind of intelligence indeed. I really doubt whether what we call "social" or

[5] On the interesting proposal to transform the sciences and the humanities from the search for knowledge to the pursuit of wisdom see: Nicholas Maxwell, *From Knowledge to Wisdom*, (London: Pentire Press, 2007).

"emotional" intelligence can ever be encapsulated by algorithms. I also doubt whether there is an algorithm for the good life. Moreover, extensive knowledge is not synonymous with wisdom either. Learning facts, facts and more facts is sometimes irrelevant in deciding which course of action we must take. It depends on our aims, not on gigabytes of information. Thus, propositional knowledge is not sufficient for guiding our lives. In order to be wise, we need to learn *how* to live well. A little philosophical reflection is enough to realize that an exponential increase in the material conditions of life at the cost of destroying the environment does not lead to a better one. Bioethics as a form of wisdom reminds us that science and technology can be only a means to the good life. Learning about the good life requires experience and practice too. Wisdom, then, shows us that quantitative knowledge is not sufficient; we need to *know-how* to live well.

There is, of course, a discussion to be had on how to enhance our wisdom. Would traditional methods such as education be sufficient or should we make, for instance, use of pharmaceuticals and other means? The debate around human enhancement such as physical improvement, psychological development, moral perfection etc. is relatively recent and much work needs to be done, especially from a critical point of view.[6] My modest contribution to this debate is here to call attention to the need to enhance wisdom as well. I do not believe that enhancing intelligence, especially the artificial form, without the wisdom of *how* to use it, is really good for us. Thus, despite the fact that I do not know of any drug to boost wisdom and even doubt whether it may be necessary, I do see clear signs that our moral concerns towards AI are only in place thanks to sensible persons such as Professor Hawking himself. That is to say, a new field in Ethics, namely *Machine Ethics*, is already being developed to discuss the values that must guide autonomous robots boosted by AI. Thus, as I will argue soon, I think that *respectful* attitudes must guide our relationships with these autonomous robots once they are fabricated. This must be the case also among artificial agents themselves: they should not be created to destroy persons (either natural or artificial). Thus, it seems clear that we have already started to find ways of placing moral constraints and limits on AI showing that Professor Hawking's prophecy may hopefully never come true.

As we humans find ways of enhancing our physical, intellectual, emotional and other capabilities and, as a result, our lifespan expands, caring, for instance for the elderly, becomes more challenging and

---

[6] On this point, see: Julian Savulescu and Norton Bostrom, *Human Enhancement*, (Oxford: Oxford University Press, 2009).

complex. We may postpone aging, but perhaps not forever and serious care will be needed at some point. Now, recent figures show that the number of carers aged 85 and over has risen in England by 128% in the last decade to around 87.000. Half of these carers work for 50 hours or more each week. Most are compromising their own wellbeing showing that we must deal with the problem in a different way to avoid aggravating it. These individuals should be cared for and not be the ones caring. An aging population imposes a greater burden on the health care system raising many issues about fairness and justice in distributing resources. In countries like Japan, where 25% of the population is over 65, caring is even becoming a social problem and some companies are turning to robots.

Consider then some examples of *caring* robots. Pepper "a robot with a heart" will be sold to care for the elderly and children. Other examples include: Wakamaru a "companion robot" designed to co-inhabit with humans; Paro a fur-covered robotic seal developed by AIST that responds to petting; Sony's AIBO robotic dog and NeCORO robotic cat covered in synthetic fur used for therapeutic purposes; Secom My Spoon an automatic feeding robot; Sanyo robot for monitoring, delivering messages and reminders about medicine; and other devices to help with the problem of caring for the elderly. To discuss one in particular, Wakamaru is a domestic robot intended to provide companionship for the elderly. It can connect to the internet and has speech recognition. One basic function is to remind the user to take her medicine. If someone falls, it calls 911. Also, in continental Europe, there are a few care giving robots in experimental testing. But are robots the best solution for caring for the elderly?

Whether robots can really perform this art depends partially on what we mean by *caring* and consequently on how we design and program them. Perhaps the most important ethical issue is what moral theory, if any, should be incorporated into programming a caring robot, for instance, a utilitarian algorithm? In "Robot Caregivers: Ethical Issues across the Human Lifespan", Jason Borenstein and Yvette Pearson discuss the issue of robots as caregivers assuming a capability approach based on human flourishing.[7] Several other questions, however, arise: will caring robots have technical abilities only or will they be designed to have feelings such as sympathy or empathy to better respond to the clients' basic needs? Should they be able to deliberate and take decisions having some degree of consciousness? Should they be capable of autonomous agency or just

[7] Jason Borenstein and Yvette Pearson, "Robot Caregivers: Ethical Issues across the Human Lifespan" in Patrick Lin *et al.* (eds.), *Robot Ethics*, (Cam., Mass/London: The MIT Press, 2012), 252f.

follow instructions blindly? If they are autonomous, should we consider them persons? Shouldn't they then have full civil rights and not just obligations? I will not be able to deal with all these questions here, but I would like to discuss further what would be the best possible *caring* robot.

First of all, let me point out some other uses we already have for robots in health care and related domains. From vacuum cleaners like Roomba to machines to wash floors, iron clothes, move objects from room to room, robots can certainly do most of the work and provide most services for elderly people at home thus improving their quality of life and wellbeing. As we saw above, robots are also designed for therapeutic purposes such as reducing stress, stimulating cognitive activities, coaching in physical therapy etc. from which the elderly can benefit. Some robots can even perform the functions of nurses such as taking blood pressure and so on. It is worth highlighting that robots are already used in other health care areas too, for example, they perform sophisticated surgeries. Moreover, caring robots may be designed for companionship, taking us for a walk, playing chess etc. A caring robot may always be willing to listen to us. It (or s/he?) may never cheat on us. In the future, they may even be the ideal companions for some of us. Anyway, there is no doubt that caring robots may improve the quality of life for everyone, including vulnerable elderly people. The possibility, however, that they become paternalistic is a real one.

How we design a caring robot becomes then a central issue for robot ethics. To shed some light on this issue, imagine we can use a *Person-o-Matic* machine to produce, by pushing some buttons, two different kinds of robot caregivers: a droid or a humanoid robot.[8] The main difference is that the droid is programmed with cutting-edge medical knowledge, has excellent caring skills etc., but always does what *it* thinks is best for you; a humanoid robot has the same knowledge and skills, but it is sensitive and open to your needs and wishes and respects your rights, especially for privacy and other basic liberties. In other words, the difference is between a mere robot caregiver and a caring robot.

Which one would you choose to take care of you if needed? I would prefer a caring humanoid robot, but I recognize that there are reasons or circumstances for someone to have a droid caregiver only (e.g., if one suffers from severe dementia). Now, it seems that we are coming closer and closer to creating such a humanoid robot and not only because of its external appearance. Consider, for instance, the recent attempts to produce

---

[8] See Steve Persons' paper "Designing People to Serve" for a use of the machine Person-o-Matic capable of making different types of artificial persons (APs). In: Lin, P. *et al.* (eds.), *Robot Ethics*, (Cam. /London: The MIT Press, 2012), 283f.

a conscious machine. Tony Prescott, a professor of cognitive neuroscience at the University of Sheffield, UK, reports progress in creating an artificial self for iCubs (the state-of-the-art humanoid robots). He remarks that sometimes he has the feeling that "someone is home" already.[9] Perhaps singularity is really near after all. Now, an iCub robot would have an ecological self (distinguishing herself from others and having a feeling of body ownership), an interpersonal self (capable of self-recognition, seeing others like herself and having empathy for others), a temporally extended self (having awareness of a personal past and future), a conceptual self (having a life story, personal goals, motivations and values) and a private self (a stream of consciousness and an inner life). Suppose, now, that you can use the *Person-o-Matic* machine and, by pushing other buttons, you could create different caring humanoid robots integrating this or that self, for instance, an ecological self, but not an interpersonal one, making up diverse robots. There are many possible combinations here. Speaking for myself, I would prefer a *caring* robot with an interpersonal self as described above. She would meet not only the conditions for personhood, but would also have moral feelings such as sympathy and empathy. Thus, if my analysis of respectful care is right and assuming that a caring robot will ever be genuinely capable of experiencing moral feelings, a humanoid caring robot capable of sympathetic concern seems to be the best possible carer.

In any case, we must give up the idea of building killer robots. We must stop creating this kind of machine: the Dragonrunner Robot; the Alpha Dog; the Predator Drone (MQ-1); Taranis; Iron Dome; Sentry Robot, etc., etc. To achieve this, we need to support the idea of reforming the UN to end wars towards perpetual peace. I would then like to point out here that a war between two or more states deploying atomic bombs is nowadays simply irrational since it may lead to the annihilation of life on this planet. This was the main concern of the so-called Cold War when global bioethics was born. The same applies to wars using chemical and biological weapons with the potential for mass destruction. Now, I get the impression that the development of "robotic wars", if they are not just electronic games, will turn out to have the same character. In other words, they will be so destructive of human life that their deployment will be irrational. What is the point of preparing for a war, say between the US and China in 50 years or so, using millions or even billions of killer robots, if it could lead to mutual destruction? Thus, I believe that we simply must "give peace a chance", not any momentary or local peace, but

[9] Tony Prescott, "The Mirror of Ourselves" (*New Scientist,* March 2015), 39.

perpetual, world peace. Thus, my suggestions to face the danger killer robots bring are: first, we all must endorse initiatives such as Human Rights Watch and call for a pre-emptive ban on *killer robots* since current warfare technology is de-personalizing and de-humanizing the killing process to such a degree that terminators will soon be not only science fiction, but perhaps our real enemies; second and in order to make effective the ban on killer robots (and indeed atomic bombs, chemical and biological weapons of mass destruction etc.) why not reform the UN Security Council and transform it into the only authority over the use of military force on earth abolishing all national armies? This is my main proposal for a new global (bio)ethics. Thus, armed drones could still be used for military purposes under such an authority, for instance to combat terrorism, but not killer robots. That is to say, armed conflicts, but certainly not wars between states, would still perhaps take place in special circumstances; however, they would not have the potential to kill millions of innocent people or even to represent an existential threat to mankind and other lifeforms. We must instead refocus our science and technology on creating caring robots. This is a central point for a global bioethics driven by philosophy.

Should caring robots be treated as persons? It seems clear that if we are, in a not too distant future, able to create such robots as described above, they will be no longer machines only, that is, a robota, a slave, an obedient servant. The best possible carer would be a humanoid robot capable of truly caring & respecting persons. In turn, she must be respected and cared for too. This may lead to human emotional attachment to caring robots and raise several other moral questions related to human-robot interactions, for instance, reciprocity of feelings etc. I see, however, nothing in principle wrong in a new world where natural (humans and other non-human animals) and artificial persons co-exist peacefully and cooperate with each other for mutual benefit. Perhaps there will exist huge differences, for instance, artificial persons would be practically immortal while humans would not, even if a human who was 100 years old appeared to be half that age by our present standards. Would that difference between immortal artificial persons and mortal enhanced humans morally matter? I don't have a clue, but one intriguing question is whether such a robot would not want to become fully human, thus experiencing mortality. This is also very singular. As we ponder about creating the best possible caring robot, we may find out that she is "just" another human being or an artificial person very much like us. One conclusion we may then reach is that the kind of care existing robots can provide is quite limited and that a truly caring person, even if artificial, is human in form.

Finally, as some robot ethicists have correctly pointed out, a major concern about robot care for the elderly is that it may replace human contact with negative consequences. Given the present stage in the development of robotics and the idea of *respectful care*, we must not regard robots as substitutes for human carers. It seems that a human and perhaps in the future a sensible artificial person must always be in the loop of care supervising robot caregivers. Robot care as provided today is very limited indeed and it is not a good substitute for human companionship. Consequently, current robots may help, but they cannot be seen as the definite solution for the problem of social exclusion of the elderly. The best we have is still respectful care as provided by responsible humans.

7.2 Holistic bioethics: *reverentia* for life

In my analysis of respectful care, I pointed out that there are many meanings attached to the words 'care' and 'respect' and I have focused on a particular context, namely when, in *special* bioethics, a scientist/doctor is looking after a subject of research/patient in a vulnerable condition while, at the same time, trying to increase scientific knowledge. I did this to make sense of the predominant use of 'bioethics', that is, to refer to the ethical problems in biomedicine and in other biological sciences despite the fact that this may be a reductionist view. Now, I also anticipated that the word 'bioethics' was first used to refer to a more general attitude, namely caring for life as a whole. In this section, I would like to go back to this initial bioethical project and to discuss this general attitude towards life, including concerns for the environment and non-human animals. As I have already anticipated, I call this project 'holistic bioethics' since it refers to an integral caring attitude towards life as a whole. My main goal is to integrate the principle of *reverence for life* into the ethical-philosophical framework of *a* common, sharable morality. I will use the word 'reverence' as a form of respect, namely of deference, but it does not have the same meaning as recognition respect. Perhaps there are only family resemblances between them.

To start with, let me recall Fritz Jahr's bioethical principle, which expands Kant's Categorical Imperative to all lifeforms, namely "Respect every living being on principle as an end in itself and treat it, if possible, as such!" According to Jahr, this principle can be found in some of both Western and Eastern philosophical traditions and in many religious practices from Francisco de Assis to Mahatma Gandhi. It leads to a general attitude of, for instance, not killing innocent humans, but also non-human animals or plants with the proviso "if possible". Its real extension is, however, unclear, but there are certainly circumstances when a person needs to kill an animal in order to save her own life. Thus, the radicalization of this principle as in some extreme forms of Jainism is not morally required by *a* common, sharable morality and may well lead to starvation and death. Therefore, by introducing a principle requiring reverence for life, this absolutizing as well as other forms of moral extremism must be avoided. Other questions, however, remain: does Jahr's principle require vegetarianism? It seems that this is also not the case since for survival reasons an Inuit may need to kill a seal to have a meal. I will return to this issue below.

To a certain extent reassembling Fritz's principle, proponents of "a land ethic" or the movement "deep ecology" have also tried to expand the moral community beyond humans. I have already mentioned Arne Naess' project of an ecosophy in the first chapter, which also calls for a new kind of wisdom, for a philosophical bioethics. Now, to quote another defender of such an approach, Aldo Leopold: "The land ethics simply enlarges the boundaries of the community to include soils, waters, plants, and animals, or collectively: the land."[10] Despite the clear implications for overcoming the anthropocentric character of most traditional ethical theories (some of which appear to have a metaphysical background taking man as made in God's image), Leopold's project seems to go far beyond what has moral significance. That is to say, a stone cannot be intrinsically valuable and has at best only instrumental value to us or to any lifeform indeed. Thus, it is too demanding to include non-alive or inanimate objects in a common, sharable morality. To be clear, however, land ethics does not lead to vegetarianism. To recognize this point, it is enough to mention Leopold's criterion for right and wrong actions: "a thing is right when it tends to preserve the integrity, stability, and beauty of the bioetic community. It is wrong when it tends otherwise."[11] Thus, hunting a hare, killing it and eating the meat does not destabilize the bioethic community. Leopold himself was a hunter and a meat eater and I do not see incoherence or hypocrisy in his views. Hunting may in some cases even be necessary to restore some balance to wildlife. What seems certain, however, is that the so called "land ethics" requires expanding *some* moral concern to life as a whole beyond humans and non-human animals. And this is not only because pollution, the extinction of species, the disruption of ecosystems, etc. have adverse economic consequences for us. This would mean treating

---

[10] Aldo Leopold, "The Land Ethic" in Michael Zimmermann *et al.* (eds), *Environmental Philosophy*, (Upper Saddle River: Pearson, 1993), 103.

[11] Aldo Leopold, "The Land Ethic" in Michael Zimmermann *et al.* (eds), *Environmental Philosophy*, (Upper Saddle River: Pearson, 1993), 106.

life as instrumentally valuable only. Life pre-existed humans and may continue without our lifeform: we must not, however, be the cause of large scale devastation and certainly we cannot deny the intrinsic worth of biotic communities with no human beings, but with other lifeforms.

From Albert Schweitzer and Aldo Leopold to more recent authors such as Arne Naess, Paul Taylor, Rolston III and many others, the intrinsic value of life was defended in the context of an environmental ethics and *respect for nature* was proposed as a fundamental principle and a primordial ethical attitude. Thus, *a* common, sharable morality may easily incorporate a principle stating such a general attitude towards life as a whole. It can be put in simple words: *revere life's inherent worth.*[12] This principle may factually not be part of *all* existing moral systems (again, we must for that reason reject the idea of *the* common morality), but it must be integrated into *a* common, sharable morality. This middle level norm may certainly lead humans to look for higher standards of conduct regarding nonhuman animals, plants and the environment as a whole. For this kind of respect, I am using the term '*reverentia*', which means a deference to life itself. It demands a special kind of respect, a general attitude of regard in the deepest sense, for life as a whole. This middle level principle can be justified by the first principle of philosophical ethics. That is to say, it is optimific, it can be universally willable and would not be rejected by a virtuous person.

This general holistic attitude is, according to some philosophers, at the bottom of special bioethics too. As Ronald Dworkin pointed out when interpreting the famous decision of the US Supreme Court about the *Roe v. Wade* case, this kind of respect for life as a whole (either conceived in evolutionary-naturalist terms or in non-naturalistic ones) may lead to an overlapping consensus among conservatives and liberals on particular issues such as abortion and euthanasia. According to Dworkin, we disagree so deeply on abortion and euthanasia because we all take so seriously the value that unites us as human beings – the inviolability of every stage of every human life.[13] We must, however, make a distinction between respecting the intrinsic worth of life and considering it sacred in a particular religious sense. It is a sign of wisdom to recognise the

[12] I provided a conceptual analysis of intrinsic value in my dissertation. I argued that Moore systematically confuses an abstract, Platonic, way of thinking about values with a much more concrete, Aristotelian, perspective, according to which intrinsic value is that which is *worth having for its own sake*. I have since used the latter conceptual framework in my bioethical works.

[13] Ronald Dworkin, *Life's Dominion*, (New York: Alfred A. Knopf. 1993), 238.

interconnections between special bioethics and *reverentia* for life as a whole, that is, with holistic bioethics.

Returning now to the examination of the principle revere life's intrinsic worth, there remains the question whether the interests of individual beings must be respected or the integrity of, let us say, organic wholes such as species, ecosystems etc. must also be. Now, since *a* common, sharable morality takes a holistic perspective, it seems clear that not only particular non-human animals can be intrinsically valued by caring for them (this is the case certainly with our pets), but also organic wholes such as entire ecosystems even if no animal lives there. Thus, the principle of reverence for life as a whole requires preserving as much existing life as we can. To recognize this, let me use a Moorean thought experiment: imagine two planets, one without any lifeforms and one with micro lifeforms even if only vegetal. It seems clear that we would value intrinsically the latter more than the former (if we valued the first intrinsically at all). Now, think of a third planet with microorganisms: it is even more valuable and so on and so forth. Our little Earth is certainly much more valuable than the previous imagined worlds. In this sense, an environmental policy based on the so called "3Rs" (reduce, reuse, recycle) may be required in mere economic, instrumental terms, but it is not incompatible with a more general respectful attitude of, for instance, preserving biodiversity as something valuable in itself. In fact, the first principle of ethics seems to require us to prioritize the first R (reduce) as an urgent *policy* to save many lifeforms here and now. In this sense, perhaps the Paris Conference on Climate Change in 2015 arrived at too little and, I hope not, too late. We must act immediately starting with more birth control to relieve the pressure on the use of natural resources, the impact on the environment, the destruction of the vital spaces of many lifeforms etc. Thus, *a* common, sharable morality gives support to life as a whole and not only to what is instrumental to our survival.

Finally, I would like to discuss briefly the use of non-human animals in scientific experimentation and for nutrition. Let me start by saying that most scientific research and teaching using animals in clinics, universities, etc. is superfluous and must urgently be stopped. There are real doubts whether teaching medicine by maltreating dogs is really needed. However, there seem also to be reasons to continue some forms of scientific experimentation without disrespecting non-human subjects. To illustrate: the search for the cure for cancer may benefit not only humans, but also non-human animals. Thus, when a non-human subject of research can benefit herself from a scientific experiment, there are no reasons not to do it, for instance, a scientific experiment using stem cells on a non-human animal to recover its ability to walk after a car accident. Here the policy also called "3Rs" (Replacement, Reduction and Refinement) can still be applied and may, giving effective priority to replacement, for instance using computer modelling etc. lead to an end of the need to use real live animals in a not too distant future. Thus, the abolition of the use of non-human animals in scientific experimentation is on the horizon in *a* common, sharable morality, but we presently still need to increase our knowledge.

The use of non-humans for sustenance is a more complex issue. There seem to be sound arguments both for and against vegetarianism. On the one hand, for a pregnant woman eating beef may be necessary to prevent health problems for her and the baby; on the other hand, most adults can live well without beef using artificial supplements such as Vitamin B12. Ethicists of different normative ethical approaches have argued in both directions. For instance, a deontologist such as Tom Regan holds that subjects-of-a-life, including non-humans, have a right to life and cannot be killed for food.[14] Peter Singer's preference-utilitarian view seems to go, for different reasons, along with this idea, namely non-human animals have an interest in living and must not be killed, despite the fact that he recognises that there are exceptions, for instance, for the Inuit.[15] However, as the Wittgensteinian philosopher Cora Diamond notes, neither of these two philosophers have presented a valid argument for not eating meat.[16] It is not immoral to eat an animal just killed by lightning in an open field. This can also be recognized when we see ethicists applying a utilitarian ethics, such as Roger Crisp does, to hold that we must in fact eat meat because it brings, if we follow a welfarist policy, more happy animals into the world maximizing in this way utility.[17] Thus, given that there is not yet agreement on this issue, *a* common, sharable morality cannot forbid eating meat. This may be recommended in particular moral systems for a variety of reasons, but cannot be enforced by public laws. Therefore, it is not morally impermissible to have an omnivorous diet. But *a* common, sharable morality must prohibit hunting for fun or other cruel sports using animals just for human delight because it represents a disrespectful attitude.

---

[14] Tom Regan, *The Case for Animal Rights*, (Berkeley: University of California Press, 2004).

[15] Peter Singer, *Animal Liberation*, (New York: HaperCollings Publishers, 2002).

[16] Cora Diamond, *The Realist Spirit*, (Cam/London: The MIT Press, 1995), 319f.

[17] Roger Crisp, "Utilitarianism and Vegetarianism" (*International Journal of Applied Philosophy*, (4)1, 1988), 41f.

The concept of respectful care may, as can be seen, be extended and applied to cover actions in holistic and global bioethics. In these domains, it has the meaning of 'reverentia' for life as a whole. In global bioethics, it seems more applicable since we are still dealing with human subjects in scientific experimentation in the international sphere. For instance, whether it is permissible for a pharmaceutical company to use human subjects in poor countries where there is no legal requirement to obtain informed consent. Respectful care forbids that. In holistic bioethics, it seems clear that we must care in a respectful manner for most non-human animals.

FINAL REMARKS

In this work, I have mainly worked out the concept of respectful care for special bioethics. I have also developed a new moral epistemology to provide solid meta-ethical foundations for it and discussed some neonatal cases to illustrate how it might work in practice. It is intended to avoid both paternalism (a danger of the Hippocratic tradition based purely on beneficence) and indifference (a problem for autonomists relying too much on individual self-determination) in dealing with scientific research involving human subjects. Without neglecting other dimensions such as global or holistic bioethics, I focused on the meta-ethical and normative basis of special bioethics trying to overcome the problems of the predominant theory, namely the four principles approach. Thus, I have argued that the intuitionist meta-ethics should be replaced with practical cognitivism in order to better know *how* to deal with bioethical cases.

To finish this book, I would like to try to sum up its main spirit in this way: care without respect is blind; respect without care is empty. The time for respectful care has come. Therefore, we must all *know-how* to *care for* a vulnerable being, that is, in a *respectful* way. This is perhaps the best lesson we can get from a philosophical bioethics based on wisdom, which has the potential to lead us into a better future.

BIBLIOGRAPHY

Aristotle. *Nicomachean Ethics* (trans. by Roger Crisp). Cambridge: Cambridge University Press, 2014.

Arras, John. "Nice Story, But so What? Narrative and Justification in Ethics." In: Jecker, Nancy *et al.* (eds.) *Bioethics. An Introduction to the History, Methods and Practice*. Sudbury: Jones and Bartlett Publishers, 2007. pp.206-225.

Arrington, Robert. "A Wittgensteinian Approach to Ethical Intuitionism". In: Stratton-Lake, Philip (ed.). *Ethical Intuitionism: Re-evaluations*. Oxford: Clarendon Press, 2002. pp.271-289.

Avineri, Shlomo and de-Shalit, Avner (eds.). *Communitarianism and Individualism*. Oxford: Oxford University Press, 1995.

Azevedo, M. A. "Health as a Clinic-Epidemilogical Concept." *Journal of Evaluation in Clinical Practice*. 21(3), 2015. pp. 265-73

Baird, Robert and Rosembaum, Stuart. (eds.) *Euthanasia: The moral issues*. Buffalo: Prometheus Books, 1989.

Baker, Gordon and Hacker, Peter. *Wittgenstein Rules, Grammar and Necessity*. Oxford: Wiley Blackwell, 2014.

Beach, Mary C. *et al.* "What does 'Respect' Mean? Exploring the Moral Obligation of Health Professionals to Respect Patients." *Journal of General Internal Medicine*. v.22, 2007. pp.692-695.

Beauchamp, Tom and Childress, James. *Principles of Biomedical Ethics* (1ªed.). Oxford: University Press, 1979.

Beauchamp, Tom and Childress, James. *Principles of Biomedical Ethics* (2ªed.). Oxford: University Press, 1983.

Beauchamp, Tom and Childress, James. *Principles of Biomedical Ethics* (3ªed.). Oxford: University Press, 1989.

Beauchamp, Tom and Childress, James. *Principles of Biomedical Ethics* (4ªed.). Oxford: University Press, 1994.

Beauchamp, Tom and Childress, James. *Principles of Biomedical Ethics* (5ªed.). Oxford: University Press, 2001.

Beauchamp, Tom and Childress, James. *Principles of Biomedical Ethics* (6ªed.). Oxford: University Press, 2009.

Beauchamp, Tom and Childress, James. *Principles of Biomedical Ethics* (7ªed.). Oxford: University Press, 2013.

Belkin, Lisa. *First, Do No Harm*. New York: Ballantine Books, 1993.

Bell, Nora (ed.). *Who Decides? Conflicts of Rights in Health Care*. Clifton: Humana Press, 1982.

Bengson, John and Moffett, Marc (eds). *Knowing how: Essays on Knowledge, Mind, and Action*. Oxford: Oxford University Press, 2012.

Borém, Aluízio *et al. Understanding Biotechnology*. Upper Saddle River, Prentice Hall, 2003.

Borenstein, Jason and Pearson, Yvette. "Robot Caregivers: Ethical Issues across the Human Lifespan." In: Lin, Patrick *et al.* (eds). *Robot Ethics. The Ethical and Social Implications of Robotics*. Cambridge, Mass./London: The MIT Press, 2012. pp.251-265.

Brink, David. *Moral Realism and the Foundations of Ethics*. Cambridge: Cambridge University Press, 1989.

Callahan, Daniel. "Bioethics as a Discipline." In: Jecker, Nancy *et al.* (eds). *Bioethics. An Introduction to the History, Methods, and Practice*. Sudbury: Jones and Bartlett Publishers, 1997. pp.17-22.

Campbell, Neil. "When Care Cannot Cure: Medical Problems in Seriously Ill Babies." In: Kuhse, Helga and Singer, Peter. (eds). *Bioethics. An Anthology*. Oxford: Blackwell, 2006. pp. 303-314.

Caplan, Arthur. *et al.* (eds.) *The Case of Terri Schiavo. Ethics at the End of Life*. New York: Prometheus Books, 2006.

Carr, David. "Knowledge in Practice." *American Philosophical Quarterly*.V.18, n.1, 1981, pp.53-61.

Charon, Rita and Montello, Martha (eds.). *Stories Matter. The Role of Narrative in Medical Ethics*. New York/London: Routledge, 2002.

Childress, James *et al.* (eds). *Belmont Revisited. Ethical Principles for Research with Human Subjects*. Washington: Georgetwon University Press, 2005.

Close, Lesley and Cartwright (eds.) *Assisted Dying. Who Makes the Final Decision? The Case for Greater Choice at the End of Life*. London: Peter Owen Publishers, 2014.

Crisp, Roger. "Utilitarianism and Vegetarianism." *International Journal of Applied Philosophy*. (4) 1, 1988. pp. 41-49.

Crisp, Roger. *Mill On Utilitarianism*. London/New York: Routledge, 1997.

Crisp, Roger and Slote, Michael (eds). *Virtue Ethics*. Oxford: Oxford University Press, 1997.

Crisp, Roger. "Treatment According to Need: Justice and the British National Health Service." In: Rhodes, Rosamond *et al.* (eds.) *Medicine and Social Justice. Essays on the Distribution of Health Care*. Oxford: Oxford University Press, 2002. pp. 134-143.

Crisp, Roger. *Reasons and the Good.* Oxford: Oxford University Press, 2006.

Crisp, Roger. *Griffin on Human Rights.* Oxford: Oxford University Press, 2014.

Crisp, Roger (ed.). *The Oxford Handbook of the History of Ethics*. Oxford: Oxford University Press, 2015.

Dall'Agnol, Darlei. "Analytic Ethics and the Morality of Universal Respect." *Cogito*. (12)3, 1998, pp. 205-210.

Dall'Agnol, Darlei. *Intrinsic Value: Analysing Moore's Ethics.* Dissertation, University of Bristol, UK, 2000.

Dall'Agnol, Darlei. "G. E. Moore." In: Demateis, Philip *et al.* (eds.) *British Philosophers 1800-2000.* New York: The Thompson Gale, 2002. pp.155-162.

Dall'Agnol, D. "What We Cannot Say, We Can and Must Speak About." In: Marek, Johann. C. and Reicher, Maria. (eds.) *Experience and Analysis*. Kichberg am Wechsel, WAB Archives, V.XII, 2004. pp. 89-91.

Dall'Agnol, Darlei. "Dworkin's Liberal Egalitarianism." *Kriterion: Revista de Filosofia.* V.2, N. 111, 2006. Online: http://socialsciences.scielo.org/pdf/s_kr/v2nse/scs_a03.pdf

Dall'Agnol, Darlei. "Kant and Wittgenstein on the Application of Rules." In: Rohden, V. *et. al.* (eds) *Akten des* X. *Internationalen Kant-Kongresses* (5v). Berlin: Walter de Gruyter, 2008a. pp.535-545.

Dall'Agnol, Darlei. "Practical Cognitivism." *ethic@ An International Journal for Moral Philosophy*. V.7, N.2. 2008b. pp.323-339.

Dall'Agnol, Darlei. "Wittgenstein and Ethical Inquiry: a Defence of Ethics as Clarification" (Review). *Notre Dame Philosophical Reviews*. 2008. Online: https://ndpr.nd.edu/recent-reviews/

Dall'Agnol, Darlei. "Themes in G. E. Moore: Ethics and Epistemology." (Review). *Mind*. v.118, 2009. pp.859-862.

Dall'Agnol, Darlei. "On the *Faktum* of Reason." In: Rauscher, Fred and Perez, Daniel (eds.). *Kant in Brazil.* New York: University of Rochester Press, v. 10. 2012a. pp. 109-126.

Dall'Agnol, Darlei. "Comments on Engelhardt's 'Beyond the Principles of Bioethics'." *ethic@ An International Journal for Moral Philosophy*. V. 11. 2012b. p. 33-36.

Dall'Agnol, Darlei. "Killing or 'Letting Die'? Conceptual Analysis and Moral Justification in Neonatal Bioethics." In: Domingues, Ivan. (ed.). *Biotechnologies and the Human Condition.* Belo Horizonte: Editora UFMG, 2012c. pp. 197-209.

Dall'Agnol, Darlei "Cuidar & Respeitar: Atitudes Fundamentais na Bioética." *Bioethikos*, 6(2). 2012d. pp.133-146.

Dall'Agnol, Darlei. "The Idealist Interpretation of Kant's Meta-Ethics." In: Tonetto, Milene *et al.* (eds). *Investigações Kantianas I*: um Debate Plural. Florianópolis: Funjab, 2012d. pp. 11-29.

Dall'Agnol, Darlei. "Pluralismo Reasonable Sin Relativismo Ético: Respuesta a Sanfélix Vidarte." *Pasajes* (València), v.42. 2013a. pp.70-79.

Dall'Agnol, Darlei. "Was Kant a Naturalist? Further Reflections on Rauscher's Idealist Meta-ethics." *Studia Kantiana*. v. 14, 2013b. pp. 141-158.

Dall'Agnol, Darlei. "Disentangling Facts and Values: an Analysis of Putnam's Pragmatic Ethics." *Principia*. v. 17, 2013c. p. 165-174.

Dall'Agnol, Darlei. "Respect for persons. Rawls' Kantian Principles." In: Dall'Agnol, Darlei and Tonetto, Milene. *Morality and Life. Kantian Perspectives in Bioethics*. Pisa: ETS, 2015a. pp.127-145.

Dall'Agnol, Darlei. "Practical Cognitivism: Knowing-how to Follow a Moral Rule." In: Kanzian, Christian *et al.* (eds) *Realism, Relativism and Constructivism.* Kichberg am Wechsel: WAB archives, 2015b. pp.53-55.

Dall'Agnol, Darlei. "Knowing-how to care." *Journal of Medical Ethics*, v.42 (3). 2016. pp. 1-6.

Daniels, Norman (ed.) *Reading Rawls. Critical Studies on Rawls' a Theory of Justice*. Stanford: Stanford University Press, 1989.

Daniels, Norman. *Just Health Care.* Cambridge: Cambridge University Press, 1995.

Daniels, Norman. *Justice and Justification.* New York: Cambridge University Press, 1996.

Darwall, Stephen. "Two Kinds of Respect." *Ethics*.V.88. 1978. pp.36-49.

Darwall, Stephen. *Impartial Reason*. Ithaca, NY: Cornell University Press, 1983.

Darwall, Stephen. *The British Moralists and The Internal 'Ought' 1640-1740*. Cambridge: Cambridge University Press, 1995.

Darwall, Stephen. *Philosophical Ethics*. Boulder, Colorado: Westview Press, 1998.

Darwall, Stephen. *Welfare and Rational Care.* Princeton/Oxford: Princeton University Press, 2004.

Darwall, Stephen. *The Second-person Standpoint. Morality, Respect and Accountability*. Cambridge/London: Harvard University Press, 2006.

Devall, Bill and Sessions, Georg. "Deep Ecology." In: Sterba, James. *Earth Ethics. Introductory Readings on Animal Rights and Environmental Ethics*. New Jersey: Prentice Hall, 2000. pp.149-157.

Diamond, Cora. *The Realist Spirit. Wittgenstein, Philosophy and the Mind*. Cambridge, Mass./London: The MIT Press, 1995.

Dillon, Robin. "Respect and Care: Toward Moral Integration." *Canadian Journal of Philosophy*. (22)1, 1992. pp. 105-132.

Donn, Steve. *Michigan Manual of Neonatal Intensive Care*. Philadelphia: Hanley and Belfus, 2003.

Downie, R. S. and Telfer, E. (1970) *Respect for persons*. New York: Schocken Books.

Downie, R. S. and Calman, Kenneth. *Healthy Respect. Ethics in Health Care*. Oxford/New York: Oxford University Press, 1994.

Duff, R. and Campbell, A. "Moral and Ethical Dilemmas in the Special-Care Nursery." In: Jecker, Nancy *et al.* (eds) *Bioethics. An Introduction to the History, Methods, and Practice*. Sudbury: Jones and Bartlett Publishers, 1997. pp. 60-69.

Dworkin, Ronald. *Taking Rights Seriously*. Cam. /Mass: Harvard University Press, 1978.

Dworkin, Ronald. *Life's Dominion. An Argument about Abortion, Euthanasia, and Individual Freedom.* New York: Alfred A. Knopf, 1993.

Dworkin, Ronald. *Justice for Hedgehogs*. Cam. /Mass and London: Harvard University Press, 2011.

Dworkin, Ronald. *Religion without God*. Cam. /Mass and London: Harvard University Press, 2013.

Elliott, Carl (ed.) *Slow Cures and Bad Philosophers. Essays on Wittgenstein, Medicine and Bioethics*. Durham/London: Duke University Press, 2001.

Emmanuel, Ezekiel and Weijer, Charles. "Protecting Communities in Research: From a New Principle to Rational Protections." In: Childress, James *et al.* (eds) *Belmont Revisited. Ethical Principles for Research with Human Subjects*. Washington: Georgetwon University Press, 2005. pp.165-183.

Emanuel, Ezekiel. "The Beginning of the End of Principlism." *Hastings Center Report*. N.25. 1995. pp.37-8.

Engelhardt, Tristram. "Ethical Issues in Aiding the Dearth of Young Children." In: Baird, Robert and Rosembaum, Stuart. (eds). *Euthanasia: the Moral Issues*. Buffalo: Prometheus Books, 1989. pp. 141-154.

Engelhardt, Tristram. *The Foundations of Bioethics* (1ªed.). Oxford: Oxford University Press, 1986.

Engelhardt, Tristram. *The Foundations of Bioethics* (2ªed.). Oxford: Oxford University Press, 1996.

Engelhardt, Tristram. *The Foundations of Christian Bioethics*. Meppel: Swets and Zeitlinger Publishers b.v. Lisse, 2000.

Engelhardt, Tristram and Jotterand, Fabrice (eds.). *The Philosophy of Medicine Reborn: a Pellegrino Reader*. Notre Dame: University of Notre Dame Press, 2008.

Engelhardt, Tristram (ed.). *Global Bioethics. The Collapse of Consensus*. Salem: MM Scrivener Press, 2006.

Engster, Daniel. *The Heart of Justice: Care Ethics and Political Theory*. Oxford: Oxford University Press, 2009.

Garrafa, Volnei. and Pessini, Leo. *Bioética: Poder e Injustiça*. São Paulo: Loyola/São Camilo, 2004.

Gert, Bernard and Culver, Charles and Clouser, Danner. *Bioethics. A Return to Fundamentals*. New York/Oxford: Oxford University Press, 1997.

Gilligan, Carol. *In a Different Voice. Phychological Theory and Women's Development*. Massachusetts: Harvard University Press, 2003.

Glock, Hans-Johann. *A Wittgenstein Dictionary*. Oxford: Blackwell, 2005.

Griffin, James. *On Human Rights*. Oxford: Oxford University Press, 2013.

Hare, Richard. *Moral Thinking: its Level, Methods, and Point*. Oxford: Oxford University Press, 1981.

Hare, Richard. "Could Kant Have Been a Utilitarian?" In: Hare, Richard. *Sorting Out Ethics*. Oxford: Clarendon Press, 2000.

Hare, Richard. *Essays on Bioethics*. Oxford: Clarendon Press, 2002.

Hart, H. L. *The Concept of Law*. Oxford: Oxford University Press, 1961.

Hayry, Heta. "Should the Decisions of Ethics Committees be Based on Community Values?" In: Kuhse, Helga and Singer, Peter. (eds.) *Bioethics. An Anthology*. Oxford: Blackwell. pp. 719-724.

Held, Virginia. *Justice and Care. Essential Readings in Feminist Ethics*. Colorado/Oxford: Westview Press, 1995.

Held, Virginia. *The Ethics of Care. Personal, Political, and Global*. New York: Oxford University Press, 2006.

Jahr, Fritz. "Bio-Ethics." In: Amir Muzur and Hans-Martin Sass (eds.) *Fritz Jahr and the Foundations of Global Bioethics*. Berlin: Lit Verlag, 2012. pp.1-4.

Jecker, Nancy *et al.* (eds.) *Bioethics. An Introduction to the History, Methods, and Practice*. Sudbury: Jones and Bartlett Publishers, 2007.

Johnson, Lawrence. *A Morally Deep World: an Essay on Moral Significance and Environmental Ethics*. Cambridge: Cambridge University Press, 1991.

Jonas, Hans. *The Imperative of Responsibility. In Search of an Ethics for the Technological Age*. Chicago: Chicago University Press, 1984.

Jonas, Hans. "Philosophical Reflections on Experimenting with Human Subjects." In: Jecker, Nancy *et al.* (eds) *Bioethics. An Introduction to the History, Methods, and Practice*. Sudbury: Jones and Bartlett Publishers, 2007. pp. 44-52.

Jonsen, Albert. *A Short History of Medical Ethics*. New York/Oxford: Oxford University Press, 2000.

Jonsen, Albert. *The Birth of Bioethics*. New York/Oxford: Oxford University Press, 2003.

Jonsen, Albert and Garland, M. (eds.) *Ethics of Newborn Intensive Care*. San Francisco/Berkeley: Health Policy Program/Institute of governmental Studies, 1976.

Jonsen, Albert. "Do No Harm: Axiom of Medical Ethics." In: Spicker, Stuart and Engelhardt, Tristram. *Philosophical and Medical Ethics: Its Nature and Significance*. Dordrecht: Reidel, 1977. pp. 27-41.

Jonsen, Albert and Toulmin, Stephen. *The Abuse of Casuistry. A History of Moral Reasoning*. Berkeley: University of California Press, 1988.

Hugher, Julian. "Ultimate Justification: Wittgenstein and Medical Ethics". *Journal of Medical Ethics*, (21), 1995, pp.25-30

Kant, Immanuel. *Practical Philosophy*. Cambridge: Cambridge University Press, 2008.

Kenner, Carole and Lott, Judy. *Comprehensive Neonatal Care. An Interdisciplinary Approach*. St. Louis/Missouri: Saunders, 2007.

Korsgaard, Christine M. "The Reasons We Can Share. An Attack on the Distinction between Agent-Relative and Agent-Neutral Value." *Social Philosophy and Policy*, 1993, 10(1).

Korsgaard, Christine. *Creating the Kingdom of Ends*. Cambridge: Cambridge University Press, 1996.

Kuhse, Helga. "Death by Non-Feeding: Not in the Baby's Best Interests", *F Med Humanit Bioeth* (1986) 7(2): 79-90.

Kuhse, Helga. *The Sanctity-of-Life Doctrine in Medicine. A Critique*. Oxford: Clarendon Press, 1987.

Kuhse, Helga and Singer, Peter (eds.) *Bioethics. An Anthology*. Oxford: Blackwell, 2006.

Kuhse, Helga. "A Modern Myth: That Letting Die is Not the Intentional Causation of Death." In: Kuhse, Helga and Singer, Peter. (eds.) *Bioethics. An Anthology*. Oxford: Blackwell, 2006. pp. 315-328.

Kuusela, Oskari and McGinn, Marie (eds.) *The Oxford Handbook of Wittgenstein*. Oxford: Oxford University Press, 2014.

Lantos, John. *The Lazarus Case. Life and Death in Neonatal Intensive Care*. Baltimore and London: The Johns Hopkins University Press, 2001.

Lantos, John and Meadow, W. *Neonatal Bioethics. The Moral Challenges of Medical Innovation*. Baltimore: The Johns Hopkins University Press, 2006.

Lantos, John and Lauderdale, Diane. *Preterm Babies, Fetal Patients and Childbearing Choices* (Cam/Mass.: The MIT Press, 2015.

Lin, Patrick *et al.* (eds). *Robot Ethics. The Ethical and Social Implications of Robotics.* London/Mass.: The MIT Press, 2012.

Lindemann, Hilde. "Context: Backward, Sideways, and Forward" In: Charon, Rita and Montello, Martha (eds.) *Stories Matter. The Role of Narrative in Medical Ethics*. New York/London: Routledge, 2002. pp.39-47.

Lindemann, Hilde. *An Invitation to Feminist Ethics.* Boston: McGraw-Hill, 2006.

Little, Margaret. "Wittgensteinian Lessons on Moral Particularism." In: Elliott, Carl. (ed.) *Slow Cures and Bad Philosophers. Essays on Wittgenstein, Medicine and Bioethics*. Durham/London: Duke University Press, 2001. pp. 161-180.

Lo, Bernard. "Behind Closed Doors: Promises and Pitfalls of Ethics Committees." In: Jecker, Nancy *et al.* (eds) *Bioethics. An Introduction to the History, Methods, and Practice*. Boston: Jones and Bartlett Publishers, 2007, pp. 236-244.

Locke, John. *Two Treatises of Government*. Cambridge: Cambridge University Press, 1994.

MacDowell, John. "Non-Cognitivism and Rule-Following." In: Holtzman, S. and Christopher, L. (ed.) *Wittgenstein: To Follow a Rule*. London: Routledge and Kegan Paul, 1981.

Macklin, Ruth. "The Inner Workings of an Ethics Committee: Latest Battle over Jehovah's Witnesses." In: Jecker, Nancy. *et al.*(eds) *Bioethics. An Introduction to the History, Methods, and Practice*. Boston: Jones and Bartlett Publishers, 2007. pp. 232-235.

MacIntyre, Alasdair. *After Virtue. A Study in Moral Theory*. London: Duckworth, 1994.

Manson, Neil and O'Neil, Onora. *Rethinking Informed Consent in Bioethics*. Cambridge: Cambridge University Press, 2007.

Maxwell, Nicholas. *From Knowledge to Wisdom. A Revolution for Science and the Humanities*. London: Pentire Press, 2007.

McLean, Sheila. *First Do No Harm. Law, Ethics and Healthcare.* Hampshire: Ashgate, 2006.

Medical Professionalism in the New Millennium: a Psysician's Charter. *Medical Journal of Australia.* V. 177, 2002. pp.263-265.

Mill, John Stuart. *Utilitarianism.* Oxford: Oxford University Press, 2001.

Mill, John Stuart. *On Liberty and Other Writings.* Cambridge: Cambridge University Press, 1994.

Miller, Franklin *et al.* (eds). *The Nature and Prospect of Bioethics. Interdisciplinary Perspectives.* New Jersey: Humana Press, 2003.

Miller, Geoffrey. *Extreme Prematurity. Practices, Bioethics, and the Law.* New York: Cambridge University Press, 2007.

Moore, Georg Edward. *Principia Ethica.* Cambridge: Cambridge University Press, 1993.

Monk, Ray. *Wittgenstein: The Duty of Genius.* London: Vintage, 1991.

Mulhall, Stephen and Swift, Adam. *Liberals and Communitarians.* Oxford: Wiley-Blackwell, 1996.

Nagel, Thomas. *The View From Nowwhere.* New York/Oxford: Oxford University Press, 1989.

Nelson, Hilde Lindemann. *Stories and theirs limits. Narrative Approaches to Bioethics.* New York: Routledge, 1997.

Nelson, James Lindemann. "'Unlike Calculating Rules'? Clinical Judgement, Formalized Decision-making, and Wittgenstein. In: Elliott, Carl. *Slow Cures and Bad Philosophers. Essays on Wittgenstein, Medicine and Bioethics.* Durham/London: Duke University Press, 2001. pp.48-69.

Noddings, Nel. *Caring. A Relational Approach to Ethics and Moral Education.* Berkeley: University of California Press, 2013.

O'Neil, Onora. *Towards Justice and Virtue. A Constructive Account of Practical Reasoning.* Cambridge: Cambridge University Press, 1996.

O'Neill, Onora. *Autonomy and Trust in Bioethics.* Cambridge: Cambridge University Press, 2002.

Parfit, Derek. *Reasons and Persons.* Oxford: Oxford University Press, 1984.

Parfit, Derek. *On What Matters* (2v.) Oxford: Oxford University Press, 2013.

Pellegrino, Edmund and Thomasma, David. *A Philosophical Basis of Medical Practice. Toward a Philosophy and Ethics of the Healing Professions.* New York/Oxford: Oxford University Press, 1981.

Pellegrino, Edmund and Thomasma, David. *For the Patient's Good. The Restoration of Beneficence in Health Care.* New York/Oxford: Oxford University Press, 1981.

Pellegrino, Edmund *et al.* (eds.) *Transcultural Dimensions in Medical Ethics*. Maryland: University Publishing Group, 1992.

Pellegrino, Edmund and Thomasma, David. *The Virtues in Medical Practice*. New York/Oxford: Oxford University Press, 1993.

Pellegrino, Edmund and Thomasma, David. *Helping and Healing. Religious Commitment in Health Care*. Washington: Georgetown University Press, 1997.

Persons, Ingmar and Savulescu, Julian. *Unfit For the Future. The Need for Moral Enhancement*. Oxford: Oxford University Press, 2014.

Persons, Steve. "Designing People to Serve." In: Lin, Patrick *et all* (eds). *Robot Ethics. The Ethical and Social Implications of Robotics*. Cam. /Mass/London: The MIT Press, 2012. pp. 283-298.

Pessini, Leo and de Barchifontaine, Christian. *Problemas Atuais de Bioética*. São Paulo: São Camilo/Edições Loyola, 2010.

Pessini, Leo *et al.* (eds.). *Ibero-American Bioethics: History and Perspectives*. Dordrecht: Springer, 2010.

Potter, Van Rensselaer. *Bioethics. Bridge to the Future*. New Jersey: Prentice-Hall, 1971.

Prescott, Tony. "The Mirror of Ourselves." *New Scientist.* March 2015.

Rachels, James. "Active and Passive Euthanasia." In: Baird, Robert and Rosembaum, Stuart. (eds.) *Euthanasia: The moral issues*. Buffalo: Prometheus Books, 1989. pp.45-60.

Rachels, James. *The Elements of Moral Philosophy*. Boston: McGraw Hill, 2007.

Railton, Peter. *Facts, Values, and Norms*. Cambridge: Cambridge University Press, 2003.

Ramsey, Paul. *The Patient as Person. Explorations in Medical Ethics*. New Haven/London: Yale University Press, 1977.

Rauscher, Fred. "Realism and Anti-Realism in Kant's Meta-Ethics: A Reply to Professor Dall'Agnol." In: Tonetto, Milene *et al.* (eds). *Investigações Kantianas I*: um Debate Plural. Florianópolis: Funjab, 2012. pp.31-43.

Rauscher, Fred. *Naturalism and Realism in Kant's Ethics*. Cambridge: Cambridge University Press, 2015.

Rawls, John. *A Theory of Justice*. Cambridge/Mass.: Harvard University Press, 1999.

Rawls, John. *Political Liberalism*. New York: Columbia University Press, 1993.

Regan, Tom. *The Case For Animal Rights*. Berkeley: University of California Press, 2004.

Reich, William (ed.) *Encyclopedia of Bioethics*. New York: Macmillan, 1995.

Resnik, David. *The Ethics of Science*. London/New York: Routledge, 1998.

Rolston III, Holmes. "Caring for Nature: From Fact to Value, From Respect to Reverence." *Zygon*, v.39. 2004. pp.277-302.

Rorty, Amélie (ed.). *Essays on Aristotle's Ethics*. Berkeley: University of California Press, 1980.

Ross, David. *The Right and the Good*. Indianapolis: Hackett, 1988.

Ross, Laine "What is Wrong with the Physician Charter of Professionalism." *The Hastings Center Report*. V. 36, n.4. 2006. pp.17-19.

Russell, Bertrand. *Philosophical Essays*. London: Allen and Unwin, 1968.

Ryle, Gilbert. *The Concept of Mind*. London: Penguin, 1990.

Savulescu, Julian *et al.* (eds.). *Enhancing Human Capacities*. Oxford: Oxford University Press, 2011.

Savulescu, Julian. "Bioethics: Why Philosophy is Essential for Progress." *Journal of Medical Ethics*, v.41, 2015. pp.28-33.

Shamon, Thomas. *An Introduction to Bioethics*. New York: Paulist Press, 1997.

Sharpe, Virginia and Faden, Alan. *Medical Harm. Historical, Conceptual and Ethical Dimensions of Iatrogenic Illness*. Cambridge: Cambridge University Press, 1998.

Scheffler, Samuel. *The Rejection of Consequentialism*. Oxford: Clarendon Press, 1992.

Schneiderman, Lawrence and Jecker, Nancy. *Wrong Medicine. Doctors, Patients and Futile Treatment*. Baltimore/London: The John Hopkins University, 1995.

Schrag, Bernard. "Social Obligation for Primary Care." In: Smith, David (ed.) *Respect and Care in Medical Ethics*. New York: University Press of America, 1984. pp. 219-272.

Singer, Peter. *Practical Ethics*. Cambridge: Cambridge University Press, 1993.

Sparks, Richard. *To Treat of Not to Treat. Bioethics and the Handicapped Newborn*. New York/Mahwah: Paulist Press, 1988.

State of Michigan, Case No. 06 1015 CZ, Answer to Complaint.

Stanley, Jason. *Know how*. Oxford: Oxford University Press, 2011.

Morrison, Eileen and Furlong, Beth. *Health Care Ethics. Critical Issues for the 21st Century*. Maryland: An Aspen Publication, 2012.

Tonetto, Milene *et al.* (eds.) *Investigações Kantianas I*: um Debate Plural. Florianópolis: Funjab, 2012.

Tooley, Michael *et al.* (eds.) *Abortion. Three Perspectives*. Oxford/New York: Oxford University Press, 2009.

Toulmin, Stephen. *The Place of Reason in Ethics*. Chicago: University of Chicago Press, 1986.

Toulmin, Stephen. "How Medicine Saved the Life of Ethics." In: Jecker, Nancy *et al.* (eds). *Bioethics. An Introduction to the History, Methods, and Practice*. Sudbury: Jones and Bartlett Publishers, 1997. pp. 25-34.

Tugendhat, Ernst. *Vorlesungen ueber Ethik*. Frankfurt am Main: Suhrkamp, 1984.

Veatch, Robert. *A Theory of Medical Ethics*. New York: Basic Books, 1981.

Veatch, Rpbert. "Hospital Ethics Committees: Is There a Role?" In: Jecker, N. *et al.* (eds) *Bioethics. An Introduction to the History, Methods, and Practice*. Boston: Jones and Bartlett Publishers, 2007. pp.226-231.

Vidarte, Vicente Sanfèlix. "Reflexiones Wittgensteinianas. Reseña del libro *Seguir Regras* de Darlei Dall'Agnol" *Pasajes*. V.40. 2012-3. pp.130-137.

Waldron, Jeremy. *Theories of Rights*. Oxford: Oxford University Press, 1995.

Warnock, Mary and Macdonald, Elizabeth. *Easeful Death. Is There a Case For Assisted Dying*? Oxford: Oxford University Press, 2008.

Widdows, Heather. *Global Ethics. An Introduction*. Durham: Acumen, 2011.

Wildes, Kevin. *Moral Acquaintances. Methodology in Bioethics*. Notre Dame: University of Notre Dame Press, 2000.

Wilkinson, Dominic. *Death or Disability*? *The 'Carmentis Machine' and Decision-Making for Critically Ill Children.* Oxford: Oxford University Press, 2013.

Williams, Bernard. *Ethics and the Limits of Philosophy*. Cambridge, MA. Harvard University Press, 1985.

Wisnewski, Jeremy. *Wittgenstein and Ethical Inquiry. A Defence of Ethics as Clarification*. London: Continuum, 2007.

Wittgenstein Ludwig. *Werkausgabe in 8 Banden*. Frankfurt am Main: Suhrkamp, 1968.

Wittgenstein, Ludwig. "Lecture on Ethics." *Philosophical Review*.V.74, 1965.

Wittgenstein, Ludwig. *Tractatus Logico-philosophicus*. London: Routledge, 1997.

Wittgenstein, Ludwig. *Philosophical Investigations*. Oxford: Blackwell, 2012.

Wittgenstein, Ludwig. *On Certainty*. New York: Harper and Row, 1972.
Wolf, Susan. *Feminism and Bioethics. Beyond Reproduction*. New York/Oxford: Oxford University Press, 1996.
Wolf, Susan. "Deconstructing Welfare: Reflections of Stephen Darwall's *Welfare and Rational Care*." *Utilitas*, Vol.18, No.4. 2006. pp. 414-426.
Zangwill, Nick. "Against Analytic Moral Functionalism." *Ratio*. XIII, 3, 2000. pp. 275-287.
Zimmerman, Michael *et al.* (eds.) *Environmental Philosophy. From Animal Rights to Radical Ecology*. Upper Saddle River: Pearson, 1993.

INDEX